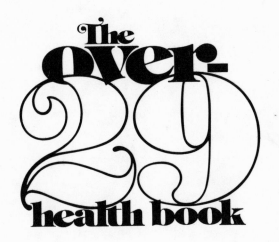

The over-29 health book

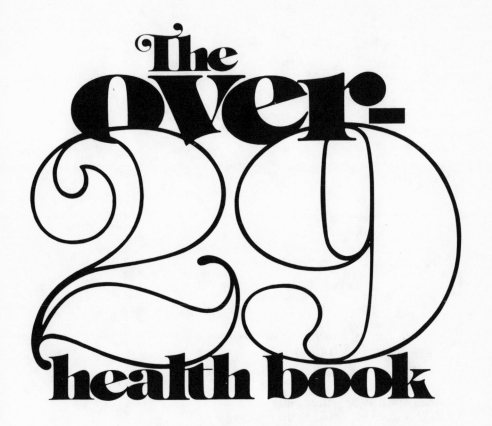

The over-29 health book

By Jeffrey Furst

DONNING
Virginia Beach, Norfolk

Cover design by Fischbach & Edenton
Virginia Beach, Virginia

The Donning Company/Publishers
5659 Virginia Beach Blvd.
Norfolk, Virginia 23502

Library of Congress Cataloging in Publication Data
Furst, Jeffrey.
    The over-29 health book.
  (Unilaw library)
  Bibliography: p.
  1. Exercise   2. Lymphatics.
  3. Middle Age— Health and hygiene.
  4. Cayce, Edgar, 1877-1945.
  I. Title.
RA781.F87   613'.04'37   79-12269
ISBN 0-915442-79-5
Printed in the United States of America
Second printing May, 1982

this book is dedicated to all
who along with me
have left our footprints
on the sands
of Virginia Beach

Contents

List of Illustrations

Acknowledgments

I wish to share here, some of my gratitude for the contributions that have been made by so many people in the course of producing this book.

First, to my publisher, Bob Friedman of Virginia Beach, who "kept the faith" and held it on his list of projects through several seasons and rewritings. Also, in retrospect to my long ago professor of Anatomy, Physiology and Kinesiology at Miami University, Dr. C. McNelly, for piquing my curiosity about the intricacies of human body functions. To artists Ray Cullis for the exercise pose drawings, and Cindy Allen for the circulatory illustrations. Special thanks to typists Pat Wortman and Jeanne Kilburn (who also publish California's *Uni-Com Guide*), also Chris Miser and particularly Darlene Swanson, who not only typed, but lent space at her Florida poolside during the first writing of the manuscript. Much critical assistance and impetus was given to shaping the final manuscript by Dr. C. Norman Shealy; Gene Mueller; my long-time favorite chiropractor, Genevieve Haller, D.C.; and favorite rolfer, Gladys Man, Ph.D.

Last, and most important, are those with whom I shared so many exercise sessions over the years. The list numbers into thousands and at the top of it would have to be Genevieve.

Other faces that reappear from the past include: John Maxey, George Dempsey, Paul Owen, Belva Hardy, Reverend Ralph Spears, Nell Clairmonte, Joel Andrews, Shirley Winston, Ted Sharp, Adelaide Crockett, Mary Ann Woodward, Ingo Swann, Beth Blasko, Ken Brock,

Vicki Greene, Mark Russell and Becky, Shirley Petersen, Don Plym, Marilyn and Bill Petersen, Marcia Moore, Frank Adams, Pat Nolan, Carol Bush, George Ritchie, Margaret Adams, Charles and Jeana Whitehouse, Joy Burton, Lew Smith, Linda Quest, Karen Buckley, Father Jim Carroll, Sister Mary, Adono Ley, Mark Thurston, Jim and Carol Baraff, Yogi Rama, Mary Jiminez, David Graham, Joe Myers, Lilli Buck, David Long, Tom and Tracy Johnson, Kay Fletcher, Blanche Berent, Ken Kansy, James Chastain, Evelyn Gordon and Mary Alice, Bob McGarey, Jean Hafford, Lorraine and Elia Lipani, Stephan Schwartz, Bob and Eileen Miller, Kay Dunlap, Lawrence Steinhart, Kathy Olander, Vi Smith, David and Caroline Freeman, Bob Krajenke, Doris House, Charlie Stevens, June Kitson, Melanie, Zelda, Tom, Kay, Gail, Dzindra, Alexandra, Meadow, Jane, Thea, Debbie, T.J., Sun Ray, Charles Thomas, Barbara, Henry, Bob, Patricia, Melody, Jim, Dan, Sid, Rufus, Bruce, Elyse, Al and Gen Mann, Fred and Maxine, The Kronicks, The Lombards, Curtis, Faith, Hope, Jim Peak, (The ancient Mariner) and _____ . (Sorry if I missed your name. Write yourself in.)

Introduction

The two greatest causes of symptoms and illness are (1) lack of exercise and (2) emotional stress brought on by the rigors of everyday life. Jeffrey Furst has dealt with the latter problem magnificently in his earlier book, *Edgar Cayce's Story of Attitudes and Emotions*. He has now rounded out the suggestions for general improvement of health by providing a comprehensive, safe and sound "lymphatic approach" to exercise, especially for those who need it most—the "over twenty-nine" age group.

I believe that if everyone would heed the advice concerning attitudes and emotions and practice the exercises that are expounded in Mr. Furst's current book faithfully, that eighty-five percent of disease symptoms would disappear. The great advantage of the exercises listed here is that they are limbering exercises which are so badly needed by the generally inactive majority of our American public. Physical exercise in itself is a terrific booster for mental health and a great assistance in simply feeling good. Also, it is well recommended herein to use your mind to help your body achieve its greatest potential, for "mind is the builder."

Whatever your occupation, whatever your activity, you can benefit by reading and using the exercise patterns and approaches to lymphatic cleansing outlined in this book.

C. Norman Shealy, M.D.

Preface

The "Over-29 exercise routine" began as a series of stretching and breathing/relaxation movements designed to meet the needs of individuals who came to week-long conferences in Virginia Beach, where they spent nearly all of their waking hours either sitting through lectures or socializing at mealtimes. Most of the conferees were over thirty to forty years old and unaccustomed to regular or vigorous exercise; but they did need some physical activity during their stay. After some thought, we put together a half-hour series of twelve exercises that required no equipment, special skills, or conditioning, and were arranged in a logical continuity as preparation for a short period of meditation which followed. Some of the exercises were variations on those recommended to specific individuals by Edgar Cayce. Some were yoga types drawn from the author's own athletic experience in coaching and teaching health and physical education.

The "Daily Dozen" as first conceived was expanded, then evolved through seven years of daily sessions at Virginia Beach and elsewhere to include several dozen exercise segments, movements and asanas. These were tested and refined, time after time during the process. Utmost emphasis was placed upon proper breathing and relaxation techniques, all designed to promote lymphatic movement and cleansing. Some movements or variations were created just for this purpose. Their continuity, too, was given careful consideration.

The "lymphatic approach" was incorporated from the start—

centering about my fascination concerning what Edgar Cayce had recommended for relaxation and lymphatic drainage of the facial and throat areas. This was accomplished by use of the "cervical release"— employing fingertip pressure to the 3rd cervical vertebra area while in a supine position. (The father of osteopathy had discovered and used the same pressure point years before Cayce, and the Orientals had known of it for centuries. Regardless of its origin or originator, it worked most effectively.) This set me to thinking about the role of lymphatic drainage and circulation in general, particularly its specific role in reducing cellular toxicity. This in turn led me on to its further relationship with the fluid dynamics and balances involved during a human body's various activities, especially during exercise.

The text which follows is the result of years of study, practice and discussions with physicians, therapists and related professionals. It will serve as an introduction to deeper implications that become all the more obvious when studying the life process, with an overview of combining exercise and our vital fluid balances. Those who have continued practicing the "Daily Dozen" routine (either in short form or fully) are unanimous in acclaiming its benefits.

My fond wish is that readers of all ages will join us in sharing the benefits of our research.

Foreword:

IN PRAISE
OF LYMPH

For some inexplicable reason there has existed to date a sad neglect concerning the role that lymphatic circulation plays in the human body's life processes, and in the difference between disease and continued well-being. Ever since Sir William Harvey first described the circulation of blood nearly four centuries ago, the role of lymph simply has never been given just recognition. (Indeed, Bartholin described and named the lymphatics just a few years later, in 1653, but who ever remembers him?) Gray's Anatomy, the classic medical text, spells out that, indeed, there is a lymphatic system, and pretty much lets it go at that—the ramifications of lymphatic circulation being left to the imagination. Certain diseases, mostly of a cancerous nature, are described by pathologists as related to lymph ducts and nodes, but these are usually regarded as transients within the lymphatic circulatory system rather than diseases of the system itself. Breast cancer, with surgical removal (mastectomy) of the afflicted mammary gland along with its associated lymph ducts and nodes, serves as an example.

Aside from such pathological considerations, there are many quite excellent books in print on the general subjects of health, holistic healing, diet, exercise, yoga, and varieties of massage or reflexology/pressure/techniques in which lymphatic circulation is scarcely mentioned (or totally ignored in most instances), despite the extreme importance of lymph in any overall assessment of optimum body functioning. *It is as if some unspeakable taboo had existed through the centuries concerning this vital portion and function within our bodies—a portion and function we can no more survive without than we can manage without food or oxygen.* Perversely, despite such relative importance, have you ever known anyone, including yourself, who has had a doctor sit down and propose a heart-to-heart chat about the function and current condition of their patient's lymphatics—or what to expect or do about this condition in the future? If the answer is yes, you are indeed a rare and privileged individual!

Among conversing friends and families, where medical parlor games are played concerning hospital/surgical costs; lengthy in-patient recoveries; with gruesome recallings of pain, anguish, suffering, expense and suspense, upsmanship demands that any casual announcement of lymph node removals or even the blockage of a major hepatic duct be topped immediately by haughty veterans of appendectomies and hysterectomies; extensive bone surgeries and traction bar suspensions; gall bladder and kidney stone removals; probes, tests, exploratories, ad infinitum. Sad, but true, even hemorrhoids, varicose veins, face lifts or nose jobs invariably receive better audience reaction than that of, say, someone's Aunt Harriet who pleads for sympathy over her recurring bouts with edema.

New Age consciousness calls for more constructive perspectives! I, for one, have come out of the closet in favor of open discussions concerning our lymphatics—and foresee the day when others such as myself will speak out boldly, without shame of prior ignorance, and proudly proclaim ourselves—in praise of lymph!

PART I

The Lymphatic Approach To Health

1 LYMPH
The Garbage
System of the Body

     The human body's composition, aside from the bones, is made up of about seventy-five to eighty percent water, the main comprising substance of all living cells. In addition to the watery protoplasm within, our body cells are constantly awash in a liquid substance, again mostly water, called "tissue fluid." Within the bloodstream this is observed as plasma, the liquid part minus blood cells. Should you skin yourself slightly, so as not to actually bleed many red cells, the clear fluid that oozes out is what we're concerned with.

     Blood plasma carries nutrients to the cells throughout the body. All necessary substances, such as glucose (blood sugar), amino acids (protein components), vitamins, minerals, antibodies, hormones and other chemical substances for regulating body activities, are suspended in this plasmic "soup"—along with blood cells and a certain amount of waste or toxic substances. (See Illustration A.) Since the blood is under pressure from the arteries, it eventually comes to capillary walls, where much of the liquid seeps through and bathes the cells with whatever it happens to be carrying at the moment. If this happens to be needed food, fine. If toxins such as alcohol or narcotics are present, the individual may become intoxicated or otherwise affected. Should more fat globules and fatty acids be carried to these areas than the body can burn up or throw off, then the fat may be stored nearby for future needs. (And, please note the less physical activity and thus the slower the circulation in any body area, all the more readily are fat components

1

A. CIRCULATORY SYSTEM

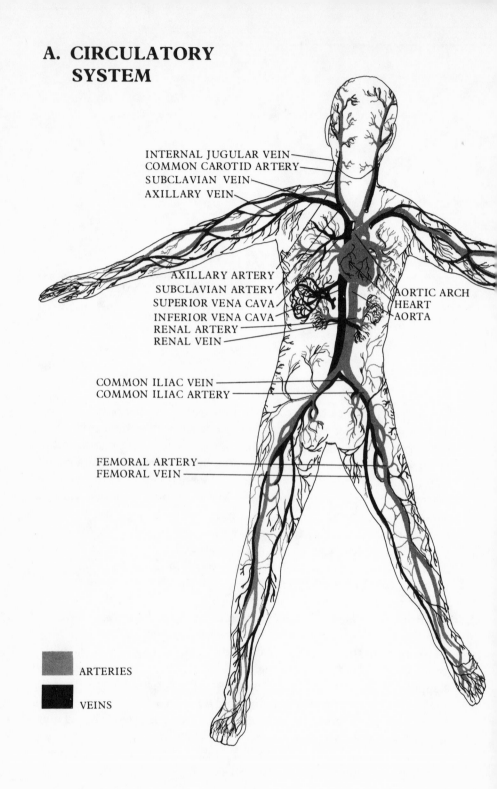

INTERNAL JUGULAR VEIN
COMMON CAROTID ARTERY
SUBCLAVIAN VEIN
AXILLARY VEIN

AXILLARY ARTERY
SUBCLAVIAN ARTERY
SUPERIOR VENA CAVA
INFERIOR VENA CAVA
RENAL ARTERY
RENAL VEIN

AORTIC ARCH
HEART
AORTA

COMMON ILIAC VEIN
COMMON ILIAC ARTERY

FEMORAL ARTERY
FEMORAL VEIN

ARTERIES

VEINS

B. HEART/LUNG/CAPILLARY SCHEMATIC

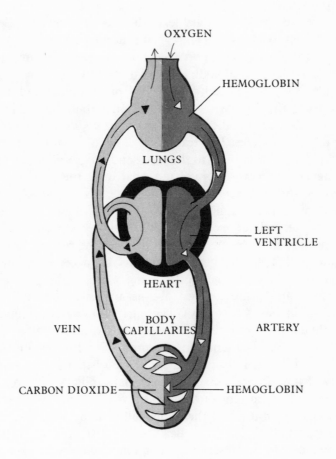

OXYGEN

HEMOGLOBIN

LUNGS

LEFT
VENTRICLE

HEART

VEIN

BODY
CAPILLARIES

ARTERY

CARBON DIOXIDE

HEMOGLOBIN

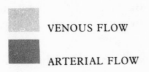

VENOUS FLOW

ARTERIAL FLOW

inclined to find a comfortable semi-permanent resting place!) Remember, too, that the capillary tubes themselves are so narrow that it takes about ten of them to equal the width of a human hair. Consequently, the red blood cells must literally line up in single file to pass through, and, obviously, if there are large amounts of fats in the diet, these substances will be pressured through the capillary walls and on to the lymphatics. (This situation will be elaborated upon in later chapters.)

Also, at the capillary level there is an exchange of oxygen (O_2) and carbon dioxide (CO_2). Oxygen is needed by the cells to metabolize (burn up) blood sugar in order to produce heat and movement. At the same time, carbon dioxide is thrown off as a waste product. Essential oxygen is carried by red blood cells from the lungs and heart through arteries to the capillaries, where in turn carbon dioxide is absorbed in solution by the blood plasma that passes by without seeping through capillary walls. (See Illustration B). This plasma, loaded with carbon dioxide, then continues to the heart and lungs where the oxygen/CO_2 exchange is reversed. Note, too, that once the arterial blood passes through the capillaries to the veins, there is considerable lowering of pressure, thus a dramatic slowing down of venous blood movement.

Meanwhile, back at the cell level (say, a muscle cell), there is a continuous interchange going on between the cell and its surrounding tissue fluid. Food, oxygen (even toxins) are accepted or rejected, while waste products are regularly being expelled as part of the cell's metabolism. As more blood plasma arrives by arterial pressure, the tissue fluid moves on to tiny collecting tubules whose function is to carry the fluid away. Once the fluid is in these lymphatic tubes or ducts, it is differentiated and identified as lymph. (See Illustration C.)

Truly, lymph acts as the garbage system of the body. Since the flow of liquid once outside the arterial capillaries is a one-way street (capillary hydrostatic pressure preventing its return), nearly all substances not used by the living cells—along with all toxins, fatigue substances (lactic acids), dead cells, nitrogenous wastes, protein substances, fatty substances (including cholesterol), bacteria, viruses, germs, etc.—must be carried away by the lymph. And, the sooner the better! Otherwise the living cells lose their efficiency, or even perish, because of their own toxic wastes. (In a sense the cells are faced with a microcosm of man's ecological problems with garbage and sewage; pollution versus fresh air, food, water, etc.)

The system of lymphatic ducts extends everywhere that the body has living cells—resembling the branches and limbs of a tree and much akin to parallel images of capillaries and veins (only much more intricate

C. LYMPHATIC
CIRCULATION

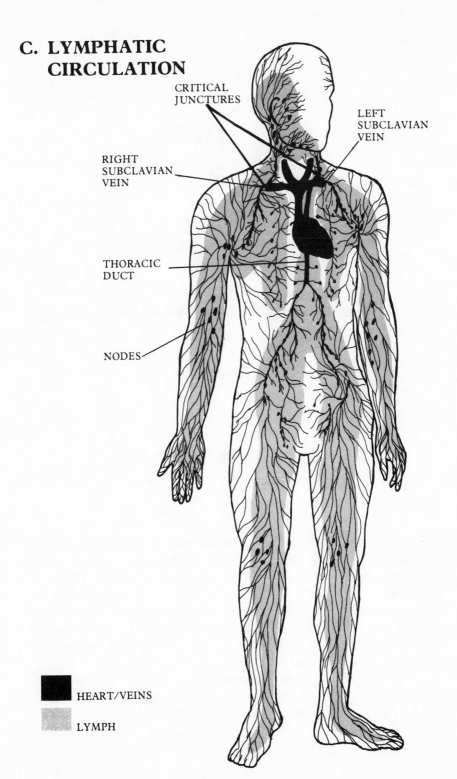

CRITICAL
JUNCTURES

LEFT
SUBCLAVIAN
VEIN

RIGHT
SUBCLAVIAN
VEIN

THORACIC
DUCT

NODES

◼ HEART/VEINS

▦ LYMPH

D. LYMPHATIC SHUNT SYSTEM

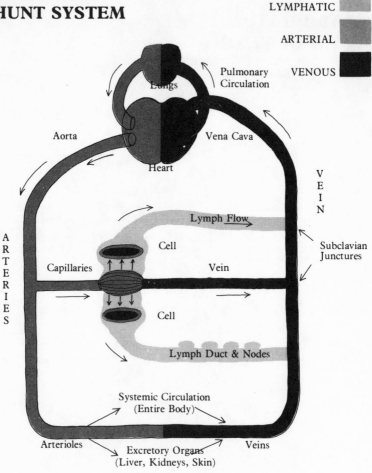

LYMPHATIC

ARTERIAL

VENOUS

Pulmonary Circulation

Lungs

Aorta

Vena Cava

Heart

V E I N

Lymph Flow

A R T E R I E S

Cell

Capillaries

Vein

Subclavian Junctures

Cell

Lymph Duct & Nodes

Systemic Circulation
(Entire Body)

Arterioles

Excretory Organs
(Liver, Kidneys, Skin)

Veins

and complex). However, once the lymph is in the lymphatic ducts, it has a problem in how it shall be propelled or moved along—away from the cells it has served—and eventually to get its load of wastes and toxins to the excretory organs. (Lungs, skin, liver and kidneys.) Basically, the system is what is known in mechanics as a shunt system. (Example: A shunt line along a railroad is a side track coming off the main line and running parallel for some distance, then switching back to the main track again.) (See Illustration D.)

In the case of our lymphatic system, all the lymph from the lower parts of the body (torso and legs) finally collects in one major (thoracic) duct that extends along inside the torso to shoulder level where it flows into the left subclavian vein (at the *angulus venosus*). Lymphatic ducts

6

from the face, head and arms also enter the subclavian veins (subclavian being "under the clavicle," or collar bone).

Once the lymph, with its supply of "garbage," flows back into the venous blood, it cycles through the excretory organs—lungs, liver, kidneys and skin—where various wastes are thrown off. Still other substances are processed, recycled and reclaimed to be used again.

Lymphatic Drainage in Relation to Exercise and Well-Being

What the systemic circulatory system conveys to living cells via blood plasma must eventually be drained away with its load of wastes (and even usable substances not immediately needed) through the lymphatic ducts—and eventually to the subclavian veins. There is a never-ending problem with lymphatic circulation—and to a lesser extent with venous circulation. Unlike arterial circulation, the lymphatics do not have their own pump. Consequently, we find there are just three ways to activate and speed up the flow of lymph away from the tissue it serves and back into the main line of pulmonary and systemic circulation. They are:

(1) *Muscular contraction:* Exercise, and—*very important* —stretching!
(2) *Massage:* Always away from the extremities and toward the spine, please! Lymph ducts have valves similar to those in veins, allowing for flow in one direction only—toward the heart.
(3) *Gravity:* Inverting—positioning the legs, arms and torso above shoulder level.

Additionally, other aspects of lymphatic flow can be problematical. A generous supply of lymph nodes are spaced along the ducts. These act as sponge-like straining stations, which can swell up and effectively stop the flow of lymph and accompanying white blood cells when certain toxins or disease-producing bacteria are present. This prevents the spread of disease, keeping inflammations or cancerous incidents localized when possible. Unfortunately, nodes and ducts can become clogged or congested with scar tissue, calcifications or fatty deposits, much as our arteries and veins do as we become more aged. Also, poor posture, inflexibility, and, again, fatty deposits (especially in the pelvis, abdomen, neck and shoulder areas) can constrict and slow the flow of lymph at its more critical and vulnerable junctions. When this happens, extremities, or finally the entire circulatory system, can be throttled and thus stagnate, producing a general toxic edema with swelling, puffiness, etc.

Then, too, there is the general condition of the capillaries and their blood supply as it relates to the lymph. If the capillaries are constricted (as with nervous hypertension or cigarette smoking), or if an individual is inactive for long periods of time, the lymph will not flow or be moved nearly enough to flush away normal waste substances. Consequently, a varying level of toxicity will exist throughout much of the body. This is why, for example, that a perfectly healthy person can be confined to bed for an extended period of time and end up feeling weak or just plain terrible. Indeed, there is some suspicion that sleeping more than six to seven hours at a stretch may be harmful to many people. (I, for one, function best with about six hours of sleep a night, plus another hour or so spent resting or napping during the day.)

Therefore, our premise and guiding principle of *The Over 29 Health Book* is that, aside from poor nutrition, *the primary cause of fatigue, disease, cell degeneration and resultant aging is poor circulation to and from (especially from) the tissues of the body, (with resulting stagnation). Living cells and organs, when continually supplied with proper nutrients and oxygen, will thrive almost indefinitely—so long as toxic waste substances are concurrently removed and regularly excreted from the body.* When we effectively move the lymph away from the cells—with muscular contraction, massage and inverting (for gravitational assistance)—we make it much easier for arterial blood to enter the capillaries and supply fresh tissue fluid, food and oxygen to the cells. This, too is the central rationale of our "over-29 exercise routine"—to effectively move and recycle the lymph and entire blood supply through the circulatory system many times over during the course of a relatively non-strenuous exercise session. In order to accomplish this we pay a good bit of attention to getting the blood moving at increased levels through the heart and lungs, plus the other excretory organs and muscle groups. (Additionally, the capillaries dilate considerably during exercise, aiding the entire cycling process.) At the same time, we concentrate on achieving flexibility and movement in the neck and shoulder areas, pelvic girdle, abdomen and spine—with added concentration on breathing, relaxation, and understanding how each exercise segment is designed to accomplish our goal of "getting out the garbage."

Lymphatic Crossroads and the Critical Junctures

One section of the body stands out above all the rest as *the most important area for consideration* in attaining maximum lymphatic movement throughout the entire body. Any perceptive student of mechanics and hydraulic principles will recognize this immediately upon scrutinizing a schematic drawing of the entire lymphatic drainage system. Indeed, it would be well for everyone to understand and keep in mind some basic facts about what makes fluids flow more readily (or be retarded), within our own internal circulatory plumbing system.

Very obviously, *if we were to plug up the main lymphatic ducts at their junctures with the subclavian veins, we would effectively block all lymphatic flow. The results would be fatal. These are the "critical junctures."* (Add to these, with slightly less emphasis, the ball and socket joint areas of shoulders and hips. See Illustration C.)

Consequently, it is our opinion that this area, which includes the upper torso, rib cage, neck, shoulders, and associated vertebrae is the most important, yet least understood, poorly attended to, or considered for attention, of any portion of the body. This opinion is based upon many years of observing practically all forms of athletics, exercise and physical training, yoga classes, dance and movement classes, massage instruction, physical therapy approaches, and relaxation techniques— as well as poring over books, manuals and articles written by most well-known practitioners in these fields. (At this point, I wish to state clearly that I am definitely not in opposition to any of the above noted forms of activity or doubt their effectiveness. Quite the contrary, they are effective in varying degrees. *And* I am convinced that if all concerned— instructors and subjects alike—were well backgrounded in awareness of the lymphatic approach and applied the principles which follow, their forms of activity would immediately become much more effective.)

So, let us consider some principles involved with movement of fluids which relate to the circulation of blood and lymph—also, the movement of air through the lungs.

E. VENTURI EFFECT

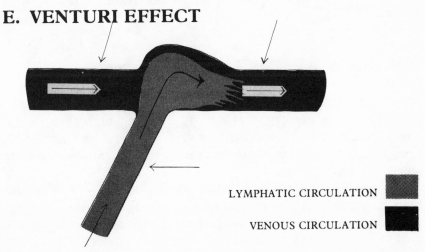

LYMPHATIC CIRCULATION

VENOUS CIRCULATION

9

First, there is gravity. It is always with us here on earth. As with rivers and streams flowing down to the sea, our internal fluids are continually influenced relative to our physical position and orientation with gravitational force.

Next, there is pressure and pressure differentials. Fluids (and air) move from high pressure/high density areas to lower areas of pressure or density. Water pouring from a garden hose or air from an electric fan are examples of this.

Pressure can be produced by pumping actions: either positive force—as with heart contractions or pumping a tire—or negative (vacuum/suction type) pumping action. Action of our diaphragm, pulling air into the lungs, is a good example of the latter. Another example, combining both actions, is a ship's propeller, which both pulls and pushes the water simultaneously as it rotates. Another variation of suction-type pumping action is achieved by what is known as the Venturi tube effect. This effect is utilized in part with many rotary impeller-type pumps—and it is the Venturi effect which aids in pulling lymph into the subclavian veins at the critical junctures. (Important fact! Keep in mind for future reference. See Illustration E.)

Pressure (and rate of velocity flow) are, in turn, affected by:

- High/low pressure differentials.
- Volume of fluid moving through an opening.
- Size (diameter) of opening (pipe, hose, tube, etc.)
- Elasticity of hose or tube.
- Bends, kinks, irregularities or protrusions in tube openings and walls.
- Viscosity (thickness or stickiness) of fluids. (If you examine blood or lymph closely, you'll find it to be quite sticky.)

Movement of Lymph at the Critical Junctures

All of the mechanical factors previously detailed are involved to greater or lesser degrees in effectively moving lymph through the critical junctures into the subclavian veins and on to the descending vena cava, from where it enters the heart's right atrium—a distance of only six to eight inches.

Additional factors interrelate in varying degrees—depending on types of physical activity such as whether a body is running, walking, swimming, sitting, standing, lying at rest or asleep. Stress situations versus relaxed states are also important considerations—as well as the influence of full or empty stomachs, and any stimulants or depressants present in the bloodstream.

Other factors are:

- Heartbeat—volume of blood flow.
- Blood pressure—condition of arteries, capillaries, and nervous system affects this (also, the venous pressure at the vena cava).
- Rate of breathing—forcible inhalation/exhalation adds suction/pressure, aiding both lymphatic and venous circulation.
- Volume/rate of venous flow through the subclavian veins (for Venturi effect).
- Pressure on the lymphatics—Muscular contraction, Gravity, Massage.
- General physical/muscular activity—speeds up circulation by placing demands on the cardio/vascular/pulmonary system.
- Water/salt/weight balance of body and bloodstream. (Dehydration can result in heat stroke, shock or other imbalances.)
- Relaxation and massage techniques (including Shiatsu, reflexology, acupressure).
- Specific mechanical relaxation of neck, upper chest and shoulder areas (cervical release, hanging, stretching—see Chapter VI.)
- Specific lymphatic pumping exercises and external pressure techniques. (See Chapter VI.)

Summary and Comments

The lymph and lymphatics are the garbage collection system of the body. The less cluttered and freely-flowing the lymphatics are, the healthier the individual will tend to be (also, the quicker to heal and faster to resolve any imbalances or diseases).

Lymphatic drainage and movement is accentuated by muscular contraction, massage and gravity. Venous blood also moves much faster under these conditions. Both are thus interrelated in the return flow of fluid volumes to the heart and lungs.

All lymph must move eventually to the upper chest/throat area before it can get back into the main bloodstream—extremely important point to keep remembering!

Exercise dilates the capillaries and allows greater quantities of blood to flow through the tissues than when the body is at rest. Increased blood flow stimulates the tissues by providing additional tissue fluid, which carries food and oxygen to the cells. (Lymph ducts also dilate considerably during exercise, providing a general flushing action.) Increased circulation, through the excretory organs (lungs, skin, kidneys, liver), aids in cleansing the blood of toxins and substances that tend to create imbalances within the body.

Capillaries may be constricted by stress, nervous hypertension, cigarette smoking or prolonged inactivity. High blood pressure also usually results in poor circulation as the smaller blood vessels constrict or narrow and increase the *resistance* to flow of blood. In each instance, lymphatic flow is reduced accordingly.

Poor circulation of the venous blood often results in varicose veins, hemorrhoids and a tendency for blood clots to form—a potentially dangerous condition. Also, as the venous circulation slows, less lymph is allowed back in at the critical subclavian junctures, which results in further general stagnation and toxicity.

The condition of a person's eyes, skin, hair, nails, breath odor and body odors (feet, armpits, etc.) are good status indicators of the condition of lymphatic circulation, toxicity and general nutrition.

The skeletal joints, with their bursae and synovial fluid, also reflect the condition of the lymph. Bursitis, dry or arthritic joints are often symptomatic of lymphatic imbalances. This is also true of the connective tissue (fascia) throughout the entire body, or in specific areas—especially at the minute (miscroscopic) cell and capillary levels.

The spinal fluid, which bathes the brain and spinal cord, is also essentially part of the lymphatic system. Its movement and replenishment are essential for a healthy central nervous system. Thus, inactivity can produce feelings of sleepiness, lethargy, dull headaches, irritability or depression.

Water that accompanies digesting foods and is drawn off from the large intestine enters the lymphatic system. Consequently, any toxic condition arising from intestinal infections or upsets, constipation, irregularity, or colonic impactions, can effect the entire body. This also holds true in the small intestine where the lacteals absorb digested food substances. (The lacteals then drain into the major hepatic ducts and on to the liver.)

The lymph and excretory organs function more efficiently when suitable quantities of water are present and being excreted. *Eight to ten glasses a day is recommended by most authorities.*

There are numerous lymphatic reflex areas about the body associated with lymph nodes which are related to various organs and muscle groups. Some of these are charted in forms of foot massage known as zone therapy. Others are well-known and utilized by osteopathic and chiropractic physicians. The practice of acupuncture, with its system of body meridians also relates to various of these reflex areas. Shiatsu and applied kinesiology techniques relate specifically to the same regions. General massage also helps in maintaining proper function and balance of the lymphatic reflex areas.

Posture, Movement and Flexibility Relative to the Critical Junctures

Prior to discussing posture and movement there are several items which are well to keep in mind regarding good health practices when we consider the ideal of a vital, healthy person. In order to be well, feel well, and function best, it is important that one:

- Stays physically and mentally active, exercises regularly, gets plenty of fresh air and oxygen.
- Practices proper nutritional guidelines (well-balanced diet).
- Has regular habits of bowel and bladder elimination; cares for lungs, skin and teeth.
- Maintains proper body weight.
- Is well-balanced in proportioning work versus rest, recreation, sleep, etc.
- Avoids excesses and extremes of food, drink, alcohol, tobacco, drugs and stimulants.
- Is mentally/emotionally perceptive and well-balanced, free of negative thought patterns, emotional hang-ups and destructive physical habits.
- Is spiritually well-oriented with one's own identity and relationship to the universe.
- Is aware and perceptive of body conditions, emotional needs, intellectual desires—and the personal responsibility involved in accepting what is, while still continually changing for the better through processes of growth, experience and understanding.

In a sense, this may seem oversimplified, since many volumes have been written concerning each facet of the above-mentioned areas of consideration. Still, in a holistic approach to life and health, all are integral and interrelated to the main theme of this chapter and should be kept in mind.

Posture

Posture in this instance pertains to the position or relative position of body parts, particularly the skeleton in relation to optimum lymphatic flow. Posture, of course, varies considerably according to whether an individual is standing, walking, running, jogging, sitting, lounging, lying down or engaged in active or semi-active sports activities—tennis versus shuffleboard, as an example.

The primary consideration concerning postural positions related to lymph flow can be centered upon the spine, pelvic girdle and shoulder girdle. So long as the spine is erect, with the hips, shoulders, head and neck kept relaxed, level and erect (in line with the spine, regardless of physical activities), there will be no pressures or impediments inflicted upon critical junctures by the skeletal parts. Also, the more often the spine is horizontal or inverted, the better the effect. Conversely, the lymphatic flow can be slowed temporarily or chronically by:

Spinal curvatures—rounded shoulders, slouching; lordosis (hollow back, pot belly); lateral curvatures affecting shoulder and hip levels.

Hollow Chest—with rounded shoulders, shallow lung capacity; usually accompanied by improper head/neck alignment and positioning.

Uneven hip, shoulder levels—caused by poor posture while sitting, standing, walking, carrying objects (purses, books, babies, etc.)

Pelvic or hip joint abnormalities, inflexibility.

Poor breathing habits—chronic shallow breathing. Inflexible rib cage, shoulders and neck.

Abdominal muscle tone—poor muscle tone affects the lymphatic flow from intestines, viscera, reproductive organs, hips and legs.

Sitting, standing, for long periods of time with little motion or change of position (long distance truck drivers or desk workers, for example).

Habitually sitting slouched, cross-legged or on one foot.

Habitually wearing tight-fitting clothing—corsets, bras,

panty girdles, support hose, stretch pants, abdominal support belts, braces, shoes or boots (even ties and collars).

Movement and Flexibility

Flexibility and body movement go hand in hand with proper lymphatic flow, particularly at the critical junctures. Assuming proper posture is being attained and maintained, it follows that the more flexible an individual is the more relaxed and free-flowing the body movements can be. This, in turn, aids in allowing lymphatic flow to move without impediments or blockages.

Flexibility, as with posture, begins with the spine, ribs, shoulder and pelvic girdles; on to the extremities—arms, legs, head—with all joints involved; including neck, jaw, knees, elbows, hands and feet. Assuming the joints are free of arthritic involvement or irregularities caused by bone/cartilage damage or impairment, any lack of flexibility can be traced: (1) Primarily, to the ligaments surrounding the joints; (2) Secondly, to the tendons which connect with muscle groups; (3) Thirdly, to the connective tissue (or fascia) which encases muscles, organs, circulatory vessels, and interlaces/interconnects them all; (4) Finally, there are other factors concerning muscle groups themselves: their general condition and tone, nerve supply, food and oxygen supply, ability to relax, stretch, and coordinate with opposing muscle groups— all important factors in relation to one's flexibility, and thus to one's movements.

Flexibility is something most individuals tend to lose as they grow older; and for the most part, it is a condition which must be maintained by regular exercises designed to produce a free range of movement and extension.

Movement is the key to both attaining/maintaining flexibility and developing proper posture habits—while at the same time providing impetus to lymphatic flow. Without movement our bodies stagnate—with movement, we flow and clear ourselves (potentially) of ever-present toxic substances. It follows that the best movements for effecting lymphatic flow are those which:

- Are free flowing, in controlled patterns.
- Entail full flexing and extension (stretching) of opposing muscle groups.
- Involve conscious breathing and relaxation techniques, both during and between exercise movements or positions.
- Incorporate movement, breathing and relaxation, centering upon the critical junctures.

Combinations of these four principles are involved within exercises which can be appropriately categorized as lymphatic pumping movements. (The specifics of lymphatic pumping techniques and the exercises best followed can be found detailed in Chapters VI and VII.)

A typical lymphatic pumping exercise entails:

(1) Alternate flexing and extension of the spine, with conscious relaxation in between.

(2) Raising of the arms, shoulders and rib cage while inhaling, followed by lowering with conscious flexing and exhalation (affecting the critical junctures and vena cava).

(3) Inverting, with head/shoulders lower than torso.

A good example is the "Good Morning" exercise, a traditional warm-up movement:

(1) Bend forward, exhaling, relax, loosen arms, neck, pull belly in.

(2) Raise up, inhaling deeply, arms overhead; head and shoulders back; up on toes, stretch.

(3) Relax forward again. (Repeat 10-12 times, or gently for several minutes if this is to be the only exercise.)

Another example known to most yoga followers would be the "Sun Salutation."

Our very best exercise for lymphatic pumping is a less strenuous variation of the Sun Salutation, which we call "The Tiger Stretch." This movement, along with proper breathing/relaxation techniques (which include abdominal vacuum, buttocks tightener and chin lock in the inverted position) combine to make it, in our opinion, the most effective single exercise one can perform for lymphatic movement. (See PART II.)

Once we have studied and learned the principles and proper techniques of breathing, flexing and relaxing in relation to posture, movement and flexibility, we will be able to incorporate such awareness in all forms of daily activities—at home, at work, or while engaged in recreational activities. The resulting benefits will be found in a free-flowing lymphatic system, a clearer head, and a healthier more effective physical body.

2 Disorders and Adverse Factors—Stress and Pain

Within a holistic approach to health, healing and preventive maintenance, there are many factors which affect the ongoing equilibrium of simple cell structures, organs, systems, or the entire body. These factors are so vitally integral to one another that no single facet can be deleted or ignored for long periods without some relative imbalance popping up—either immediately or on a long-term basis. Take diet as an example and consider the long-range effects of deleting an adequate supply of a simple substance such as calcium or Vitamin C from one's food intake. A deficiency disease results—with ultimate deterioration of the skeletal system, teeth, and debilatory effects upon the muscles and connective tissues. The entire organism ends up out of balance, diseased, because of one single dietary factor. Such examples could be essayed or detailed without end. However, it is not within the intent or scope of our book to explore fully all the ramifications of the factors which follow, mostly in outline form. Suffice to say that from a holistic approach, the following disorders and adverse factors will relate in obvious fashion:

Sluggish circulation in general:
    (1) Inactivity, sedentary occupations, lack of exercise.
    (2) Poor posture, inflexibility at critical junctures.
    (3) Poor circulation from heart/lung conditions, which can cause:
        a. Congestive heart disease or emphysema—resulting in edema, poor lung function.

b. High blood pressure—hypertension/arteriosclerosis.
(4) Overweight—fatty impediments throughout the body, throttling the circulatory system.
(5) Endocrine gland imbalances, especially high/low thyroid or adrenals.
(6) Blockages—"clogged plumbing" resulting from scar tissue, calcifications, infections, postural/bodyweight problems.
(7) Deficiency diseases or imbalances resulting in lethargy, listlessness, low blood pressure, premature aging, loss of hair, teeth, sexual/reproductive incompetency.

Toxicity resulting from:
(1) Improper diet, indigestion, acid/alkaline imbalances, improper fluid intake and balance—vitamin/mineral deficiencies.
(2) Malfunctions or infections affecting excretory organs (liver, kidneys, lungs, skin, mucous membranes).
(3) Infections or irregularity of the digestive tract and/or reproductive systems.
(4) Teeth, gum, or joint infections.
(5) Allergy reactions to food, drugs, environmental conditions, pollen, etc.
(6) Alcohol or drug abuse.
(7) Accidental or knowing intake of toxic materials with food, water or environmental/occupational contacts.
(8) Carcinogens, irritants in general, residual toxins (asbestos, lead, mercury, etc.).
(9) Lack of oxygen; high carbon monoxide levels.
(10) Blood deficiencies and chemical imbalances.

Adverse effects of cigarette smoking:
(1) Capillary restriction—accentuates aging/skin wrinkling, mucous membrane problems.
(2) Carbon monoxide factor (anemia effect). Displaces essential oxygen.
(3) Emphysema-lung/capillary damage.
(4) Carcinogens—lungs, throat, mouth, tongue.
(5) Hypoglycemic syndrome—adrenal/pancreas damage, preliminary to diabetes.

Adverse effects of excessive alcohol intake:
(1) Damage to liver, kidneys, brain, nervous system.

    (2) Alterations of personality, energy/productive levels, self-esteem.

    (3) Poor nutrition, usually.

Long-term adverse circulatory effects upon:

    (1) Skeletal system:
- a. Arthritis, swelling, deformation, bone spurs and calcification.
- b. Bursitis.
- c. Rheumatism.
- d. Softening/deterioration of bones and cartilage.
- e. Hardening of the fascia (calcifications).
- f. Accelerated aging.

    (2) Muscular/fascial systems:
- a. Dryness of ligaments and tendons.
- b. Loss of movement/flexibility; pain and irritation.
- c. Loss of muscle tone and strength.
- d. Postural changes—drooping of head, shoulders, ("Dowager's Hump" syndrome).
- e. Hardening of the fascia (calcifications).
- f. Accelerated aging.

    (3) Nervous system:
- a. Sensory deprivation or loss of:
  - a. Hearing.
  - b. Sight.
  - c. Smell and taste.
- b. Balance and coordination.
- c. Mental alertness and memory—personality.
- d. Motor abilities affecting:
  - a. Walking.
  - b. Talking.
  - c. Driving vehicles.
  - d. Mechanical tasks.
- e. Nervous tics or tremors.
- f. Imbalances as noted through attention to acupuncture meridians and zone therapy sensitivity.
- g. Senility.

    (4) Circulatory system:
- a. High blood pressure leading to nervous hypertension, arteriosclerosis (hardening of the arteries), capillary restrictions, aging, potential aneurisms and strokes (arterial breakdowns), added work load on heart, congestive heart disease or coronary occlusions.

b. Low blood pressure, leading to edema (swelling), potential blood clots (Thrombosis).
c. Infections to veins (Phlebitis).
d. Varicose veins, hemorrhoids (valve incompetency).
e. Heart—Damage to valves, pericardium, or nerve/impulse regulation centers.
f. Bloodstream, leading to anemia and toxemia, lowered resistance to infections.
g. Capillaries easily broken or bruised, slow to heal, adhesions, scarring, calcifications.

Stress

"Stress is unquestionably the major health problem in the world today," declares Dr. Hans Selye, a world authority on stress. "It's a killer!" He adds, "Medical research has demonstrated beyond a doubt that stress causes ulcers, heart attacks, hypertension, migraine headaches and mental illness." Other experts are agreed that *stress is a contributing psychological factor leading to cancer* and is also held responsible for aging, arthritis, colitis and being accident prone.

So what is stress? By definition: "Stress is the non-specific response of the body to any demand made upon it." (Conclusion: We will never be without stress!) The experts differentiate between *"dis-stress"*—resulting in nervousness, irritability, insomnia, inability to concentrate, anger, or loss of muscle control—and *"pleasant," "happy"* or *"beneficial"* stress. (Stress without distress is the idea.) Happy stress, for example, could be elicited when someone special gives you a warm embrace and lingering kiss—or the team you've rooted for all season comes from behind in the closing minutes of a crucial game and wins!

Whether with distress or happy stress, regardless of cause, the results are similar. The body responds with an increase in heart rate and change in breathing patterns. Most often, body posture or "body language" will reflect whether the individual has reacted with distress or pleasantly to a situation. Consider the changes in stress and body language that might well take place if your team loses at the buzzer! (Distress! Loud vocalizing! Arm waving! Recriminations to the officials! Loss of a bet, yet!)

Our lymphatic circulation is *always under stress*—foods digesting, muscles pumping blood and pressuring air through lungs—every movement presents a minor stress involvement on muscles, nerves, joints and ligaments. The key and solution, of course, is to continually flow through life without reacting with distress to stressful situations. Again, various factors are involved and interrelated—nutrition, environmental conditions, one's mental/emotional/spiritual condition, levels of health and vitality, biorhythm cycles, age and experience, self-integration/confidence, intelligence, and finally the ability to accept and flow with the here and now; also, holding an attitude/awareness of being personally responsible for one's own actions/reactions to the "is-ness" of whatever situation may arise is important.

Distress is the body's reaction to sudden demands, inner conflicts, irritating, tension-producing addictions, fears, anxieties, expectations, external social pressures or restraints, and long-term inability to resolve and accept one's experiences as they have occurred.

As a contrast to negative occurrences, some peak stress situations relate to experiences which are quite pleasing, exhilarating, uplifting and profoundly meaningful.

The difference, as noted by Edgar Cayce*, is that distress (such as anger, anxiety, jealousy, hatred, etc.) actually produces poisonous/toxic substances which must be carried off and cleansed from the lymphatics. Contrarily, he noted that loving/positive attitudes and emotions such as during peak uplifting experiences did just the opposite—producing harmonious healing energies and substances throughout the body. (Consider childhood situations—tears and tantrums versus giggles and sheer joy.) In effect, *we make ourselves sick*, and by the same token we can choose to make ourselves well by constructively controlling the attitudes we hold and the emotions we express. (The annals of psychic/spiritual healing are filled with cases of individuals healed of serious long-term impairments during an uplifting emotional or spiritual experience.)

*See *Edgar Cayce's Story of Attitudes and Emotions.*

Pain and Discomfort

Pain and pain syndromes are probably the best examples of a body's reaction to stress. Whether a hurt is physical, mental, emotional, or even spiritual, physically real or psychosomatically induced, the body is found to be under stress. Short-term pain syndromes are beneficial in alerting the body to the fact that something is apparently wrong and needs attention. (If no more than a fly or mosquito bite begging to be rubbed and the offender chased off.)

Long-term pain is another matter. A person with arthritis or serious spinal problems will often have obvious, near-continual, physically-induced, pain problems. In cases of more serious mental/emotional imbalances, with chronic headaches, anxiety attacks, deep depression and insomnia, along with allied aches and pains, irritability and nervousness, the presence of stress is also readily apparent. However, many deeper aspects of personal experiences include actual traumas, fears or fantasies, which contribute to such distress symptoms, yet are usually multi-faceted, complicated and not simplistically uprooted and eliminated.

However, in practically all such cases it can be noted that the individual is concurrently either in a state of endrocine imbalance, overall toxicity, or experiencing improper levels of blood chemistry (possibly anemic, hypoglycemic, mineral/vitamin deficient, etc.). It can also be noted that in most instances there will often be a history of poor nutrition, extensive drug usage (prescription or other), extensive body weight fluctuation, chronic cigarette or alcohol addiction, back/shoulder/neck/pelvic problems, poor eliminations, and lack of regular exercise. Observing this from the lymphatic viewpoint, it is quite obvious that all too many adverse factors have ganged-up on these individuals—to a point where they are overloaded with imbalances tearing them in different directions, while at the same time the lymphatics and excretory organs are unable to make proper headway against additional toxic materials being manufactured by the process of pain and emotional distress itself. Pain and suffering merely create further distress as the individual body literally poisons itself with its own self-perpetuating negativity.

3 Vitality, Health and Healing

"Vitality is the level at which the life force expresses itself."

Health can be defined as, "that quality of life which enables one to live most and serve best in personal and social relationships." Energy/vitality levels move in cycles and patterns. Biorhythm charts are one method of observing such levels (physical, mental, emotional) and seem to be applicable for many individuals.

The following are essentials for maintaining vitality and health or promoting healing (readers will note various areas which may need personal attention):

Water—as pure and fresh as obtainable. Most authorities recommend six to ten glasses per day—more if physically active or in warm environments.

Fresh Air—daily. Accompanied by conscious deep breathing.

Daily Exercise—a brisk walk with deep breathing is fine for starters. Preferably one would follow the "over 29" exercise routine. Ideally one should have the heart/lung capacity and perseverance to "Puff/Pant/Perspire" daily. (That is, exercising to the point of fairly heavy breathing and perspiration.)

Balanced Diet—with proper digestion and assimilation. Avoid animal fats; pork, beef, processed meats; junk food, sweets; foods with additives and preservatives.

Proper Vitamin/Mineral Intake and Balance—consider

supplements, especially those recommended for combating stress (B-complex, C, E, Pantothenic acid, folic acid, lecithin, brewer's yeast). Many of the herb teas also can aid one's overall well-being (Ginseng, for example).

Proper Bodyweight Range—for one's age, height, bone structure and general activities. (Should any sudden fluctuation in weight occur for unknown reasons, or if contemplating a diet with weight loss in excess of ten percent of one's bodyweight. See your physician for consultations.)

Properly Functioning Excretory Organs—and care of same. In addition to the lungs, liver, kidneys and skin, the mucous membranes, teeth, gums and hair require regular attention. This also holds true for the genital organs.

Regular Bowel and Bladder Evacuations—Edgar Cayce's readings recommend that everyone should have periodic colonic irrigations and noted that many cases of general toxicity stemmed from fecal impactions associated with diverticulitis or chronic constipation. Plenty of water, plus bran and acidophilus in the diet will help—plus the exercises in our "Daily Dozen" routine. (Also, it has been waggishly noted that "Modesty has ruined more kidneys than bad alcohol." Possibly!)

Proper Functioning and Balance of the Endocrine Glands—Edgar Cayce noted, as have other mystics, that most of the endocrines are closely associated with the chakras, or spiritual centers of the body (seven in number, they relate to the seven tones of the musical scale, also the seven colors of the spectrum). Exercise tends to stimulate them and bring them into closer harmony. Color and sound can also be used as therapeutic balancing agents.

Properly Functioning Nervous System—plus a well-balanced mental/emotional flow in reaction to demands and stress situations placed upon the body.

Effective Circulation—sufficient heart/lung capacity to handle demands from exertion such as jogging or swimming. (All blood vessels and lymph vessels should be open and free-flowing.) Bloodstream properly supplied with proportionate cells and essential nutrients.

Balanced Activities—properly proportioned amounts of work versus recreation; sleep, study, creative expression; attention to home, family, community or other activities.

Intelligence—more than just capacity for knowledge and ability to understand relationships, intelligence is "that quality of mind which endows its occupant with relative levels of awareness of consequence" (my definition—J.F.). Of course experience and education plus ability to think or reason are factors in "awareness of consequence," yet they themselves grow at the same time their contribution stimulates added wisdom or growing awarenesses of consequence. So there is another factor, or quality of mind, whether we call it being simply bright, wise, smart, or even a genius—it does manifest itself in ways that are often not discernible when using traditional I.Q. tests. My rationale here is that the mind builds both to and with its level of awareness of consequence—in direct relationship to what is held in consciousness as its ideal. And there is more involved here than simply conscious mind. The mind of man is much more complex than even the brain. (Consider the brain as an extension of our minds rather than the opposite.)

So—consider as an ideal a fully functioning, tuned in, balanced, lymphatic system within your body. After that, everything and anything that can possibly affect your body and your body's continued well-being will be viewed by a part of your mind's scanning system as relating to lymphatic circulation. Lymph in turn relates to everything concerning your body—its structure, its functionings, its balances or imbalances. The consequences are endless. Therefore, it follows that the lymphatic approach is a very simple, intelligent (awareness of consequence) approach to health, healing, exercise and well-being.

Approaches to Lymphatic Cleansing

There are several areas which should be noted relating to cleansing or "purification" of the body which, in turn, affect toxic levels within the lymphatics. Colonics have been mentioned previously in the chapter and are recommended, especially for individuals who are hospitalized, bed-ridden, paraplegic, or suffering from diverticulitis or chronic constipation.

Baths, Saunas—alternate hot/cold treatments in hot tubs, steam baths or Jacuzzi-type pools are very good for stimulating and cleansing the skin and lungs. When possible, aromatic oils can be added with beneficial results for the lungs. (Caution is advised for sauna or steam room users—avoid over-dehydration or strain upon the heart.)

Packs and Inhalants—various aromatic oils and other items are effective when used as inhalants, rubs, or packs— mentholatum, eucalyptus, wintergreen, etc. The Cayce files recommend numerous substances and applications in these areas. (See book references.) Among them was a general recommendation for epsom salt packs or baths for arthritis and castor oil packs (external) for numerous intestinal, liver and kidney difficulties.

Cleansing Diets—a typical cleansing diet is one which passes a fair amount of bulk material and water through the intestinal tract; provides a minimum of nourishment, absent of fats, proteins or starches—allowing the digestive organs a respite—and concurrently takes a load off the excretory organs, particularly liver and kidneys. Since the liver and kidneys are the primary organs involved in maintaining the body's water/mineral balances and acid/alkaline balances, these important functions are allowed to stabilize during the cleansing period. The kidneys throw off acid in the form of urea or uric acid—the liver throws off alkalines in the form of bile, which in turn neutralizes stomach acids and homogenizes fats as food enters the intestinal tract from the stomach. This area, the duodenum, is also where pancreatic enzymes are interjected for digestion of proteins, sugars and starches. Further along in the small intestine, the digested foods, now in solution, are absorbed into the lacteals and moved on to the liver via the major hepatic ducts. From there, they are metered into the bloodstream.

Note: The bloodstream itself maintains a very specific, limited-range, acid/alkaline balance (ph) at all times. Therefore, it is a misnomer to refer to the blood itself as being too acid or too alkaline. Imbalances show up outside the blood stream through the lymphatics (as in the above-mentioned lacteals and hepatic ducts), skin, breath, saliva, stomach (acids), urine, and feces.

The typical cleansing diet may last anywhere from three days to a week and generally entails eating various fresh fruits or raw vegetables, or the juices of same. (No salt, spices or seasonings. Herb teas are OK.) Some diet examples are:

Grapefruit Diet—all you can eat for several days. (This may not agree with some bodies which react unfavorably to citrus or are too alkaline to begin with.)

Grape Diet—all varieties. Same rule as above. Drink plenty of water, too.

Banana Diet—use fully ripened fruit. (Also consider that bananas contain a fair amount of fat.)

Vegetable Diet—combinations of all the raw carrots, celery, green onions, green peppers, cucumbers, parsley, water cress, greens, sprouts, beets and ripe tomatoes as available; interspersed with juice from same passed through a blender. (A small amount of fresh lemon or lime juice, garlic, or apple cider vinegar is OK for seasoning.) After three days, it is fine to begin cooking some of the combinations, if the diet is to be continued for a longer period. Add more onions and garlic, tomatoes or asparagus to cooked portions. Very good for bloodstream and circulatory vessels. Canned tomatoes are OK, especially those with no preservatives.

"Delicious" Apple Diet—this was an Edgar Cayce recommendation for a number of people, and one of my own personal favorites. All the Red or Golden Delicious apples you care to eat for three days, the more the better. Herb tea is OK. Plenty of water if one tends to become constipated, though the usual trend is otherwise.

Note: In all the above-mentioned diets it is well to follow a practice used in Cayce's Apple Diet. After or during the second day, include a daily dosage of one to two tablespoons of olive oil (more, if constipation is noticed). This stimulates the liver to evacuate the gall bladder of its bile, so you may feel a bit bilious afterward—but you will definitely find that you will be "Getting out the garbage."

Juice Diets—various fruit or vegetable juices can be utilized. Take as much as one cares to. Some individuals will do well to avoid a total citrus or tomato juice intake (it affects acidity/alkalinity). Before going on juices alone, it is well to have thoroughly cleaned out the colon via colonics or one of the fruit or vegetable cleansing diets. If juices are continued for long periods, it is also well to consider colonics or enemas later on. (I remember one occasion when the colonic machine operator related that the person before me had been relieved of a fair quantity of barium—this despite the fact that the person's last barium intake was *two years prior* as part of a series of Gastro-intestinal tests!)

Vegetable Juice—combinations as noted before. Check the health food stores and juice bars for ideas.

Concord Grape Juice—a favorite. Best diluted to taste with some water.

Apple Juice—natural, unfiltered, unsweetened preferably.

Grape/Grapefruit/Papaya Combination—this is also one of my favorites. An excellent energy picker-upper or as an adjunct to reducing bodyweight. Proportions are: one 46-ounce can of unsweetened pink grapefruit juice: one 46-ounce can or jar of unsweetened grape juice; juice of three to four lemons; two cups of papaya concentrate; two quarts of water. Mix together and refrigerate.

Fasting—there is much to be recommended in adapting short fasting periods to one's dietary patterns. Many have found that a one-day fast each week is very beneficial. Usually, only water or juice is taken for a 24-36-hour period.

Caution! Longer fasts, however, present certain problems.

As the body begins breaking down its own reserves of fats and proteins, a number of toxic substances are thrown off into the lymphatic circulation and must be eliminated. These include not only fatty acids and urea, but also any number of trace elements originally ingested and stored as part of the fat and protein molecules. As with the computer logic of "garbage in: garbage out," this can present difficulties for individuals who have long ingested large quantities of drugs, animal fats and foods with preservatives, additives, sodium derivatives and metallic traces of lead, copper, mercury, arsenic or the like. Consequently, it is very foolhardy to jump into a prolonged fast without proper preparation—which includes consulting with a physician well-versed in nutrition and weight-loss diets and one who will have the appropriate laboratory tests taken both before and during the fasting period. (This also holds true for weight-loss programs where one intends to drop over ten per cent of one's bodyweight—especially so for anyone attempting weight loss via liquid protein intake only. *No one with a history of kidney or liver problems should embark on a liquid protein weight loss diet without careful consultation and ongoing analysis by a qualified medical doctor.* In general a liquid protein fast requires large intakes of water to cleanse the kidneys and specific mineral/vitamin supplements to offset body essentials being depleted during the catabolic "ketosis" process.) The toxic releases which occur during long-term fasts can result in serious psychological disturbances and altered states of consciousness. While one person may perhaps become illuminated or saintly, partly as a result of continued fasting, others may end up disoriented or in mental institutions.

Weight Loss and Weight Control—Weight loss entails a degree of cleansing, but should be approached with caution as with any form of fasting. There are any number of popular approaches expounded by best-selling authors or groups (such as *Weight Watchers*) who have carved out their particular niche. Most of these are biologically sound so long as the individual is in good health to begin with. The best one for you is the one that works—while at the same time not throwing your endocrines or psyche (or whatever) out of balance in the process. (Also avoid being a "rebounder" who goes back to old food patterns once the desired weight level is attained. Those old fat cells just love to fill up again at the earliest opportunity.)

We would also note the advantages of being aware of stress factors which often cause individuals to react by reverting to old patterns of behavior—patterns that often include compulsive eating and drinking of the same kind of caloric combinations which produced the overweight situation in the first place. Also, cravings or compulsive food binges are usually centered upon the worst possible foods—often the very ones that a person is basically allergic to.

The Lymphatic Approach to Weight Control Suggests:

(1) Twelve weeks of balanced activities—daily exercise, fresh air, sunshine, cleansing diets (each month) followed by a well-balanced intake of food, vitamins and minerals (stress formulas, especially).

(2) Elimination of: Animal fats (butter is OK), high-cholesterol meats; pork, beef (fish, fowl, lamb, veal, with skin and fat removed, are OK); processed sugar; starches; junk foods; commercial ice cream and dairy products, carbonated beverages, alcohol. Reduction of habits or addictions leading to toxicity. (Smoking, sweets, pastries, heavily-spiced foods, etc.)

(3) Attention to posture, flexibility and critical junctures.

(4) Attention to excretory organs and eliminations. (Consider adding bran and acidophilus to the diet. Plenty of water, too.)

(5) Thorough study and understanding of the anatomy, physiology and ramifications of the lymphatic approach.

(6) After twelve weeks of daily exercise, along with the dietary recommendations, changes will be observed. Since exercise normalizes the body, some measurements and body portions will have changed in size, though the weight may have remained much the same. (Or a person may have gained or lost some weight in the very direction they wanted without any concerted, conscious effort.) By then, the body will be well-conditioned and balanced nutritionally to a point where it can handle a planned weight loss regimen without getting thrown out of balance or seriously depleted in the process.

(7) The more effective weight-loss/weight control diets recommend:

a. High protein/low fat intakes. Organic meats, fish, fowl (avoid pork and beef), vegetable proteins, fresh fruits and vegetables.

b. Elimination of salt and sodium derivatives.

c. Elimination of sugars, starches, alcohol.

d. Plenty of water with proper vitamin and mineral supplements. (A popular combination capsule contains lecithin, kelp, apple cider vinegar and B-6.)

    e. Regular exercise; fresh air and sunshine.

    f. Changes in attitudes and habit patterns regarding food, drink and one's dependency upon them.

External Approaches to Lymphatic Movement and Cleansing

A certain parallel can be drawn between external lymphatic pumping movements and those used in emergency first aid situations, where a victim's heart beat and breathing have stopped. Artificial respiration (as with mouth-to-mouth resuscitation) has been used successfully for a number of years in restoring breathing. Only recently however has the technique of hand pressure pumping of the heart itself gained widespread attention as a device to keep a cardiac arrest victim's blood circulating to the brain until the heart muscle can be electrically stimulated and its beating action restored. Alternate pressure and relaxation on the person's chest and upper abdomen will effectively send blood flowing through the heart's chambers in sufficient quantities to keep the brain cells from deteriorating due to lack of oxygen. (In hospital/surgical cases, the heart may be exposed and literally hand-pumped by attending surgeons.)

In similar fashion, one's lymphatic circulation can be stimulated in the upper chest and abdominal areas (thus, at the critical juncture areas and pulmonary regions) by proper alternate hand pressure and relaxation, tied in with the subject's own breathing and body movements. Such basic thoracic pumping movements as we are about to describe can be applied by a masseur, therapist, physician, or friend, in situations where subjects have lung/throat/abdominal congestion and are unable to perform physical exercises or otherwise exert themselves.

Lymphatic Pumping and Drainage

All of these should be preceded by the "Cervical Release." That is, hand/finger pressure held firmly at the third certical vertebra junctions for two to four minutes. (See Chapter VI, #10.)

    (1) *The Thoracic/Lymphatic Hand Pump.*

        a. Subject lies on back, knees bent, hands to sides, on floor or firm pad.

        b. Operator kneels at head level, places palms on subject's upper chest, thumbs just under the collar bones, fingers widespread.

c. Subject exhales fully as operator applies firm pressure to the upper rib cage. (Hold exhaled breath for a count of three.)

d. Subject inhales as deeply as possible, raising arms overhead and stretching. Operator removes hands as inhalation begins, grasps subject's bent knees and presses them firmly to the subject's chest. (Both hold pressure, inhaled, for a count of three.)

e. Both release. Subject, exhaling, brings knees and arms back to their original position. Operator again presses hands on subject's chest for full exhalation.

f. Repeat twelve to fifteen repetitions, or more if desired. (An extremely weak subject may need assistance on the knee movements.)

Note: Full inhalation and exhalation with the pressure held between for the full three counts is extremely important. It is the alternate pressure and relaxation that gives extra impetus to lymphatic movement (also to the pulmonary circulation).

(2) *The Abdominal/Lymphatic Hand Pump.*

a. Subject again lies on back as above.

b. Operator kneels to one side facing subject's knees, places hands palms down at base of subject's rib cage. On subject's exhalation the operator applies firm pressure to the abdomen while sliding hands slowly down the abdomen to the thighs. (Oil is recommended.) Subject holds exhalation for 3-4 counts.

c. Subject inhales as deeply as possible, raising arms overhead and stretching. Operator removes hands as exhalation begins, grasps subject's bent knees and presses them up firmly to the subject's chest. (Both hold on inhaled pressure for a count of three.)

d. Both release. Subject, exhaling, brings knees and arms back to original position. Operator repeats sliding pressure movement upon subject's abdomen.

e. Repeat twelve to fifteen repetitions, or more if desired. Operator may want to switch to the other side part way through. (Again, a weak subject may need assistance on the knee movements.)

Note: Again, full inhalation and exhalation with proper pressure technique is very important. *Caution!* Do not do this on a full stomach, or if there are evidences of any internal infections or other complications. (Gall stones, kidney stones, intestinal blockages, hernias, etc.)

 (3) *Breathing Techniques (Pranayama).*
   a. Bellows breathing can be very effective in improving circulation, cleansing the lungs, and raising energy levels.

    This is done seated, spine straight and erect, abdomen/diaphragm relaxed. Breath is forcibly expelled by rapid abdominal contractions. (Through the nose.) No inhalation attempt is required, as the air returns when the abdomen relaxes. Contractions and relaxations are repeated as quickly as possible, twenty to fifty repetitions.

   b. Alternate nostril breathing is advocated for balancing the chakras and possibly one's yin-yang aspects. Various techniques are employed. (See recommended yoga books in Appendix.)

 (4) *Lymphatic Pumping Exercises.*

   Most of the exercises detailed in the next chapter were selected because of their effectiveness in moving the lymph.

   The best of these are incorporated in proper continuity within "The Short Routine." Best of all is "The Tiger Stretch" (with abdominal vacuum and buttocks tightener).

 (5) *Inverting Gravity Techniques.*
   a. Slant boards.
   b. Inclined exercise areas.
   c. Hanging bars for loosening shoulders and neck.
   d. Sitting, resting while inverted.

 (6) *Massage Techniques.*
   a. Self massage. (See PART II.)
   b. Subject/Operator massage.
   c. Mechanical devices, hand-held types; belt vibrators; roller machines; water pulsation types.
   d. Sensual massage using aromatic oils, music,

incense, color, soft touch or slow hand movements with feathers, hair, soft cloth, blowing air, patting, stroking, etc.

e. Polarity massage using reflexology/acupressure principles in aligning energy imbalances, yin-yang, etc.

f. Auric massage. Similar to polarity theories, though practitioners usually lean more toward spiritual or psychic healing as their rationale.

g. Healing hands (laying on of hands). Some individuals are well-documented for being channels of healing when touching or massaging others. Theories vary from psychosomatic (faith healing) reversals and divine spiritual intercession, to alterations of intersecting (thus, attuning) force fields between healer and subject.

(7) *Relaxation, balancing/attuning techniques.* Release of stress, tension or imbalances invariably results in heightened lymphatic movement and lowering of toxic levels.

a. The Third Cervical Release for lymphatic drainage (See Chapter VI, #10)

b. Meditation

c. Biofeedback

d. Autogenics

e. Hypnosis

f. Reflexology

g. Acupressure

h. Do-In, Shiatsu

i. Acupuncture

j. Music, color therapies

k. Singing, chanting, dancing

(8) *Cleansing Techniques.*

a. Diets, fasting (for liver, kidneys, skin).

b. Colonics, (for colon, intestines).

c. Steam baths, saunas (for lungs, skin).

d. Packs, (sand/mud packs; epsom salts, castor oil).

e. Rubs (olive oil, almond oil, lanolin, castor oil—for sore ailing joints).

f. Inhalants, (menthol, eucalyptus, turpentine, Cayce-apple brandy keg).

g. Tonics, herbs, cell salts.

h. Treatment of mucosity (Glyco-Thymoline, colonics). (See—cleansing in *Integral Yoga Hatha*, by Swami Satchidananda.)

i. Chelation. Entails treatment for removing toxic metals, such as lead, mercury, arsenic, etc., from the body. Diagnosis and therapy by a qualified physician is necessary for such therapy.

Note: A great number of items recommended by Edgar Cayce and their applications are available through the Cayce materials. Contact: The Edgar Cayce Foundation, Association for Research and Enlightenment, Box 595, Virginia Beach, Va. 23451. For health products recommended by Edgar Cayce (available items and price list) contact: The Heritage Store, P.O. Box 444-B, Virginia Beach, Va. 23458. (804) 428-0100.

(9) *Structural Alignment.*

a. **Chiropractic**—Entails manipulation and adjustment of the spinal vertebrae and appendages, primarily to relieve pressure and nerve imbalance at the various articulations or joints. Basically, hand pressure is used by the practitioner.

The art has evolved in recent decades as with most therapeutic approaches. The modern, updated chiropractic physician often employs muscle testing, applied kinesiology, reflexology, pressure techniques, packs, rubs, dietary diagnosis and diet recommendations. X-ray observations of the spine, pelvis and shoulder girdles often pinpoint areas that are in need of specific adjustments or long-term corrective therapies. Corrective exercises and manipulation, even cranial adjustments are being found most effective in many cases.

b. **Osteopathy**—deals also with the skeletal system and its attachments. However, the osteopath is a medical doctor, thus licensed to prescribe drugs and administer same. Some also perform orthopedic surgery. In general, osteopaths employ hand techniques leaning more toward reflexology and pressure releases than the basic spinal adjustments or manipulations employed by chiropractic physicians. There is a certain degree of similarity in approaches by practitioners of both professions aside from the administering of drugs or performing surgical procedures.

c. **Physical Therapy**—employs various approaches for individuals with birth defects, growth impairments, partial paralysis or diseases affecting skeletal structure, posture and movement. Treatments center on halting the inroads or existing deteriorations, and employing corrective exercises; often swimming and pool exercises; traction or operative procedures, followed by healing/therapy periods involving casts, braces, or other devices.

The lymphatic approach suggests special attention be given these individuals in regard to lymphatic movement and cleansing.

d. **Structural Integration**—known as "Rolfing," Structural Integration was conceived and developed by Dr. Ida Rolf, Ph.D., who initiated her studies from a background in Biochemistry and Human Psychology. Rolfing approaches structural alignment from the standpoint of major fascia areas of the body (connective tissues) and their relationship to gravity, posture alignment and balance. Individual treatment consists of ten sessions, each requiring about an hour, spaced usually a week apart. Some subjects eventually desire additional advanced sessions for specific problem areas.

The great advantage of Rolfing is that the body changes effected are relatively permanent. That is, the subject will seldom revert to old misalignments so long as proper attention is given to exercise, posture, movement and flexibility afterward. With this in mind, an offshoot of Structural Integration known as "Patterning" has been developed as a follow-up to (or even in lieu of) Rolfing. The greatest clamor concerning Rolfing arises from tales of pain and discomfort related by persons who have been Rolfed. (Or persons who knew someone who was Rolfed!) This is an individual subjective experience relative to the subject's sensitivity or pain thresholds and the practitioner's technique.

Note: I can speak personally concerning this, since I have been Rolfed—and I received a great amount of favorable physical changes as a result; relief of long-term low back, pelvic and shoulder stresses—far surmounting whatever pain and discomfort I experienced in the process. As a result of my personal experience and acquaintance with numerous persons who have been Rolfed, I highly recommend the procedure for anyone who can find a Rolfer and pay the price. (It isn't cheap—$40-50 per session, and there aren't nearly enough qualified practitioners available).

e. **Consciousness Techniques**—assuming we accept or entertain as a viable premise Edgar Cayce's statements concerning negative thought forms creating toxic imbalances or circulatory restrictions, then we can well approach lymphatic cleansing from the standpoint of "Consciousness Cleansing." There is considerable evidence to support both this premise and the worthwhile overall health and healing aspects affected by consciousness expansion or consciousness changes formulated by various holistic healing groups and humanistic psychological approaches. Basically, most of these follow a rationale somewhat similar to this:

- Personal acceptance of full responsibility for one's own present being—physically, mentally and emotionally.
- Acceptance of one's previous faults, failures, inadequacies and shortcomings (accepting/eliminating guilt feelings, regrets, etc.).
- Acceptance of one's own present condition—physically/mentally/emotionally—as basically OK and subject to new experience, growth and change.
- Recognition of suffering, stress and upsets caused by old prior formed addictions, habits, demands or expectations centered upon self's preoccupations, or self's dependency upon and reactions to others, and carried over to the present.

- Elimination of such consciousness-dominating addictions, habits, demands and expectations by means of processes in re-cognition/re-programming techniques. These entail varying forms of subjective experiential exercises; interaction with others; attaining understanding of relationships and self and others from the standpoint of open-ness, honesty, compassion, love and forgiveness.
- Fully awakening to a sense of oneness of all creation and appreciation of the diversity of creation's infinite patterns and relationships (especially human ones), rather than feelings of separation, inadequacy, avoidance or repulsion.
- Fully accepting the Is-ness of everything surrounding (or within) one's sphere of awareness (good/bad, right/wrong, should/shouldn't, yin/yang, old/young, life/death, birth/burial, summer/winter, laughter/tears, pain/pleasure, joy/sorrow, highs and lows).
- Moving in consciousness and within relationships according to one's inner guidance—in regard to mental/emotional ideals, spiritual purposes and evolving lifestyle or patterns of activity.
- Loving, accepting others as they are, for what they are, allowing them to be what they care to be (rather than expecting them to fill roles or models of our own making).
- Living fully, joyously, in the spontaneity of the Here and Now—and the surprising banquet of life that each new day thrusts before us. Having faith and acceptance that the Universe prepared it just for us—for our own experience and understanding.

PART II

The "Over 29" Exercise Program

4 Preparation and Training

It would probably be simpler to write an entire book on training than to attempt condensing all the worthwhile thoughts and suggestions available into one chapter. Besides, it's much more important that you *do* the routine and get started at learning how it affects your body and your outlook—rather than sitting around and contemplating upon how you *would* do it if you ever got around to doing it! So whatever you do— begin right away!

Physical Surroundings—All you need is enough room to lie down or stand up with your arms and legs fully extended. On hard surfaces a pad, rug or blanket is advised. Seek all the fresh air and sunlight available. Inside, keep room temperatures down. At home a pleasantly decorated room with a scenic view is preferable. Soft music may help in setting the mood, but it should not be so loud as to distract your concentration. Smells are important too—flowers and incense often help.

Clothing—The exercise should be done barefoot with as little clothing as possible. Whatever is worn should be comfortable and not bind or restrict movement. Leotards or bikinis are fine for women. Sweat suits or elastic stretch type exercise clothes are also good to have available for outdoor exercising, or when first warming up.

Time of Day—I personally prefer to exercise around sunrise. My second choice is early evening in lieu of eating. Whatever one's desired choice, or whatever hour is chosen for practical reasons, it is best to be consistent and stick close to the same time of day every day. This is especially true while making the routine part of your life during the first twelve weeks. Weekends may tend to change your schedule, but try not to let a weekend pass without making this daily investment toward the health of your body.

Partners or Groups—Some people find that solitary exercise, along with meditation, is very satisfying after they've worked at it for a time. Others prefer a partner or group. However, don't let the lack of a group or absence of an exercise "buddy" serve as your excuse for not starting or continuing with the exercises. One of the most worthwhile benefits you'll receive from this program is the personal satisfaction of having continued the discipline for twelve weeks of daily sessions— truly a growth experience in itself for those who adhere to it.

Concerning Goals—The first goal, of course, is to complete the initial twelve-week series and in the process learn to do the various exercises and poses to the best of your ability. (And don't stop altogether just because you miss a few days for some reason—start all over again.) At the end of your first exercise quarter we suggest you take time to give some consideration to both long range and short range personal goals.

But for the most part don't worry or concern yourself about such matters until you've satisfied yourself that you are capable of doing that one main and simple thing that you've set out to do, which is to do the routine, daily, for a dozen weeks (or at least do some of the exercises daily).

Obviously there must be a desire for better health and appearance, and the willingness to agree with the statement that, "Our bodies are our best investment."

No one can exercise for you, or especially make you want to, other than you. Your decision therefore is your own. Whether you decide to continue on, in whole or in part, or drop it along the way, is your prerogative. Either way, do it with no particular amount of regret or remorse.

Self Examination—Very few people are totally pleased with their bodyweight and/or physical proportions and capabilities. Most all of us would prefer to be either somewhat taller, or thinner, or be larger or smaller in certain areas, etc. Even those who are well proportioned and maintain an ideal bodyweight usually would like to have more energy, stamina, flexibility, will-power, emotional control, or the like.

We suggest that after the initial twelve weeks of exercise you take time to seriously examine yourself, with the thought of setting both short and long range goals for yourself. A word of caution here: don't go overboard on goal setting or even attempt to make decisions as to goals until you've thoroughly examined where you are in relation to where you may wish to be—The price you might have to pay could be heavier than you find yourself willing to endure for very long. Goals should be determined as within reason and based on previous experience and attainments, otherwise there may be too much discouragement for an individual to maintain the self-discipline necessary to see things through. So start with goals that are relatively attainable in a short period of time in order to get into the habit of accomplishing what you set out to do, unless you are well accustomed to achieving whatever you have determined to achieve. No small item this. In fact we could well include it at the head of our self-examination list—which we recommend that you do.

Which of the following areas do you feel a need to improve upon?
(1) Bodyweight, dietary considerations.
(2) Proportions in general, measurements in particular?
(3) Energy, vitality. (Also ability to bounce back to normal after strenuous or fatiguing activity.)
(4) Strength, endurance, heart/lung competency.
(5) Flexibility (specific areas)?
(6) Body conditioning, muscle tone, coordination, agility, speed, quickness.
(7) Lung capacity.
(8) Posture, spinal alignment.
(9) Circulation, skin condition; ability to stand temperature extremes; cold hands, feet, etc. (include blood pressure, pulse).
(10) Digestion and elimination (include teeth & gums).
(11) Emotional stress or nervous tension (anxieties, fears).
(12) Amount and quality of relaxation and sleep (also time periods).
(13) Sexual competency.
(14) Eyesight.
(15) Willpower, discipline.
(16) Mental alertness, memory, learning ability.
(17) Concentration, meditation.
(18) Eliminating bad habits, addictions.
(19) General health, feeling of well being; resistance to common diseases, colds, etc.
(20) Other?

Setting Goals—Make a priority list one through twenty and assign each of the areas a number according to what you feel should be their relative importance in an overall perspective (both long and short range) particularly in regard to what is considered the foremost area or areas in need of immediate improvement. (In case of ties or strong preferences, place them side by side.)

Are the top priority items areas which you are capable of working on and improving consistent with your needs, desires and past accomplishments? For example, if you need to lose weight and want to, have you ever really reduced successfully before? If so, will you do it again in the same manner? Perhaps better? Or, if you've never had success before, what could you do this time that would succeed when what you tried previously didn't work? (Considering that latter possibility, such items should not be taken as top priority challenges or disciplines unless there is a very strong personal desire and committment to move and change a previously stubborn obstacle or habit patterns.)

Now you are ready to write down which of your priorities are to receive special concentration during the next twelve-week period. *Do it!*

Following Through—"Nothing succeeds like success." As you continue with the exercises you will find your ability to perform the exercises continually improving and your self-confidence will grow too—usually in direct proportion to the concentrated effort that you've applied. There is one very human pitfall which often shows up here. We have a strong tendency to throw ourselves wholeheartedly into the poses and exercises that we do well and not give proper attention to the ones which are difficult or painful. *Avoid getting overbalanced in any direction.* Set aside extra practice time and concentrate on exercises you perform with the least flexibility, comfort or finesse. Work on your weak points at these other times in addition to extra concentration during the regular sessions, and before long you'll find that all the weak spots have disappeared and in their place is a very well balanced and more confident you!

Peaks, Pain and Body Cycles—Our bodies are never the same from one day to the next, so don't be overly chagrined when your body goes through its customary up and down cycles of physical/mental/ emotional highs and lows. Get to know and accept yourself in all extremes and extremities. There are times for all of us when it seems that we'll just never make any further progress in some of the stretching poses. Then, for no apparent reason, a previously difficult pose or painful extension quietly relaxes and falls into place. (Ah! Is this not happiness!) The time for utmost personal progress is when we are experiencing peaks of energy levels, concentration, and success in relaxing the areas that hinder flexibility. It is often well to extend oneself longer and with more determination when experiencing these peak periods if time is available. For example, you may hold a pose longer or repeat it another time in order to properly set an imprint in your body's memory mechanism that you really did it—and thus, can do it again!

A certain amount of discomfort is something we must learn to accept when striving for more flexibility. We didn't get to our various states of rigidity, inflexibility and misalignment overnight—rather they are the sum total of an entire lifetime. Naturally, the body resists when we attempt to prod it out of its old self-satisfied ways. The body rejects mechanical changes with pain. And if we submit to pain's siren song the body may triumph and keep right on controlling us, rather than we ourselves controlling our bodies. Aside from the customary stiffness and soreness during the first week or two of exercise you should experience only a small amount of stiffness later on—when first exercising, before you get properly moving and warmed up, or when sitting or resting in one position for an extended time. *Incidentally, the parts that hurt the most will usually indicate exactly where you need the most work!*

Most of the discomfort experienced in stretching exercises is caused by muscles, tendons and ligaments being stretched beyond their customary limits—and especially by their inability to relax and allow themselves to lengthen to the extensions desired. A young mechanically sound human body can assume many very extreme flexed postures and extensions within a fairly short period of training. (Witness the Olympic gymnasts and their ages.) However, most "beyond twenty-niners" have lost much of that youthful flexibility (if ever we had it!). The amount of flexibility we attain with the routine will hinge to a great extent on how limber we were in our youth and how long it has been since we maintained a fair level of flexibility and activity. So don't expect to become a human pretzel in twelve easy lessons, just move along at your own pace, in your own good time. The only one you are comparing with is your own body; so learn how to tell it to relax and in so doing the discomfort of resistance will gradually subside. (Concentrate, mentally focusing upon specific areas that give you trouble, as with the hamstrings and lower back and tell them, on each exhalation to relax! relax! relax!)

Hanging Bars and Incline Boards—Everyone should have these available. Adjustable chinning bars can be set in any convenient doorway and used several times a day to stretch the shoulders and upper dorsal vertebrae. This helps to align and straighten the spine, release neck tensions, raise the rib cage and strengthen the shoulders, hands and arms. All you need do is hang with head tilted slightly down for several seconds. (Chin ups are not necessary.) A few slight up and down tugs will help the stretch. (Good to do just before beginning the exercises.)

With what you now understand of the lymphatic circulation, the advantages of an incline board should be obvious. It is fine to just rest upon one, head down, for relaxation. Once or twice a day is recommended, or more if you find the effects immediately beneficial. (Women will also find this helpful during their menstrual periods or during pregnancy.) Anywhere up to fifteen minutes at a time should be sufficient.

5 The Routines and Exercises

As noted previously, this exercise program was developed to fit the needs of most individuals, especially those beyond age thirty to forty or those unaccustomed to regular exercise. It requires no equipment or special skills. At the same time, it is quite worthwhile for individuals of all ages who desire a basic activity ideal for physical well-being, body conditioning and/or preparation to meditation.

Some of the exercises are familiar yoga types, some are from the author's own experience in athletics, health and physical education. By design, they have been placed in a continuity which is physiologically sound and purposeful. The "Daily Dozen" was evolved through years of daily sessions by thousands of participants at Virginia Beach and elsewhere. Those who have continued with the routine are unanimous in acclaiming its benefits.

We suggest you give it a full try—daily for a dozen weeks—(hence the current title). After twelve weeks you may want to vary some aspects of the activity according to your own individual physical situation. Fine, but give the basic routine time to sink in.

The
Routines

The "Daily Dozen" Extended Routine
(Takes about one hour to complete)

(1) "GOOD MORNING" EXERCISE
(2) JANGLE
(3) SHOULDER SHRUGS
(4) ARM AND LEG CIRCLES
(5) KNEE BENDS ON TOES
(6) "BARNYARD SHUFFLE" LOOSENER
(7) HIP CIRCLES (HULA HOOP)
(8) FORWARD BENDS (KNEES BENT)
(9) EGG ROLL
(10) CERVICAL RELEASE
(11) KNEE AND ELBOW TOUCH
(12) SHOULDER STAND
(13) THE BRIDGE (OR "WHEEL")
(14) THE FISH
(15) LEG RAISES AND SIDE STRETCH
(16) THE CAMEL AND PELVIC STRETCH
(17) SUPINE LAYOUT
(18) THE COBRA
(19) THE LOCUST
(20) THE BOAT
(21) THE BOW

(Break: Having thoroughly arched the spine and exercised the muscle groups involved, we are now ready to move on to some less strenuous loosening activities in a seated position. Now is the time to get up and move around for a minute or two, should you desire to do so.)

(22) YOGA MUDRA (SEATED) AND BELLOWS BREATHING
(23) SHOULDER LOOSENER AND "BALINESE DANCER" MOVEMENT
(24) FACE AND SCALP MASSAGE
(25) ELBOW SQUEEZE
(26) CHEST AND SHOULDER MASSAGE
(27) GROIN AND PELVIC LOOSENING— "STRAIGHT ARROW," BUTTOCKS ROCK, BUTTERFLY, FOOT MASSAGE, GROIN STRETCH MOVEMENTS

(28) JANGLE (PALMS UP)
(29) FLAT-FOOTED SQUATS
(30) KNEE AND GROIN STRENGTHENER
(31) THE CROW
(32) ALTERNATE SIDE BEND AND TOE TOUCH
(33) TIGER STRETCH (WITH VACUUM AND
BUTTOCKS TIGHTENER)

The "Daily Dozen" Short Routine
(Takes about one-half hour to complete)

The short routine is for beginners who are not conditioned physically for the entire routine, or when not enough time is available to complete everything. (The number of repetitions should be determined by the participant according to time and energy available.) Instructions for each exercise follows in Chapter VI.

(1) "GOOD MORNING" EXERCISE
(2) JANGLE
(3) ARM AND LEG CIRCLES
(4) KNEE BENDS (ON TOES)
(5) HULA HOOP
(6) EGG ROLL
(7) CERVICAL RELEASE
(8) KNEE AND ELBOW TOUCH
(9) SHOULDER STAND (OR "THE FISH")
(10) "CAMEL" WITH PELVIC STRETCH (OR
SIDE STRETCH)
(11) REPEAT JANGLE, FLAT FOOTED SQUATS
(12) TIGER STRETCH

The "Daily Dozen": Short Short Routine
(Ten to fifteen minutes to complete)

(1) "GOOD MORNING" EXERCISE
(2) JANGLE
(3) EGG ROLL
(4) CERVICAL RELEASE
(5) TIGER STRETCH

Note: These two pages are repeated at the end of the book as a tear-out for easy reference.

The Exercises

Caution: The extended routine should be taken on slowly and patiently, as a learning process, unless you have a well qualified instructor assisting you, or if you've already had a good bit of yoga training. Better to do the Short Routine well as a beginning and each day add another exercise or two, taking time to concentrate fully on the newer movements (especially the breathing and relaxation segments). By the end of twelve weeks you should be able to run through the entire series. (When short on time, it would be best to delete the foot massage and/or facial massage segments as they take up several minutes of the routine.)

Note: Should you desire to add a spiritual aspect, we suggest you begin with this affirmation: "Father/Mother God, I will that this activity creates in me a greater channel that thy will be done."

I. "GOOD MORNING" EXERCISE

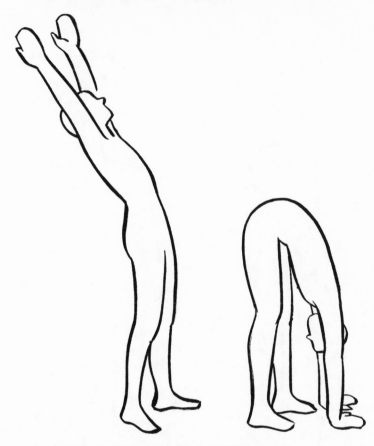

A. Stand with feet shoulder-width apart.
B. Bend forward in a relaxed manner, exhaling and
   loosening the shoulders, neck, and hands.
C. Raise up and stretch while inhaling deeply, head up,
   back arched, on tip toes.

Repeat seven times. This is a well-known traditional
stretching exercise which was also recommended by Edgar
Cayce for a number of people. Its advantage is in
stimulating breathing and circulation as a warm-up at the
beginning of our routine.

   Balance may be difficult at first when raising on toes.
Concentrate on looking at a specific spot on wall or ceiling. If raising on
toes is bothersome for you, remain flat footed during this exercise.
(Advanced students may wish to begin here with the Sun Salutation
rather than this simple form of stretching.)

II. "JANGLE"

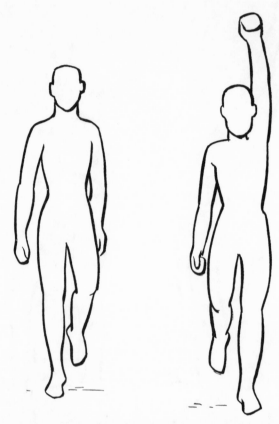

A. Jog in place while loosening the shoulders, neck, hands and lower extremities. Continue until breathing is well-accelerated.
B. Alternately raise the arms overhead (still jogging) and stretch, making a clenched fist.
C. Inhale deeply, holding each clenched fist at the top for several running steps. Repeat five to ten times with each hand. (Concentrate on deep inhalation.)

This is an excellent warm-up exercise. It stimulates circulation and breathing while loosening the muscles and joints. The stretching in turn helps to align the spinal column and firms up the underarms, chest and shoulders.

Concentrate on relaxation during first part. Make like a "Rag Doll." *Inhalation during all exercises should be through the nose!* Exhaling through nose or mouth is optional, though nose exhalation is preferable.

III. SHOULDER SHRUGS

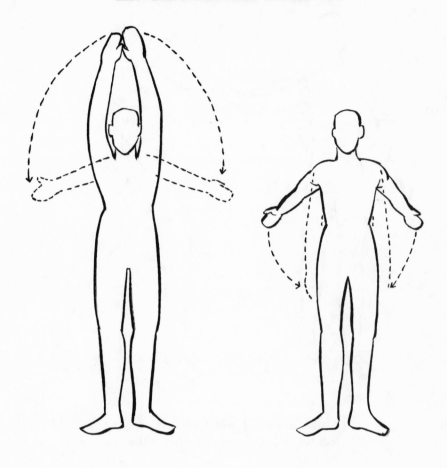

A Raise the arms forward and shoulders up, then arms overhead, continuing through in a complete circle. Repeat seven to twelve repetitions.

B. Reverse the motion and circle back seven to twelve times.

Breathe in as you raise the shoulders. Shoulders should touch the ears! This exercise is useful for improving posture and flexibility of the shoulder girdle. It is used here to loosen the areas under the collar bones and upper ribs where the lymphatic ducts drain into the venous circulation. (Most important!)

IV. ARM & LEG CIRCLES

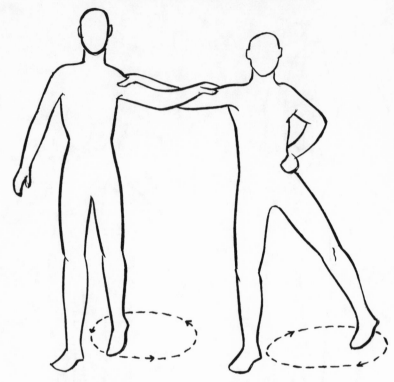

A. Legs

1. Stand on left leg while holding on to a firm object for balance (not necessary if you have good balance).
2. Extend right leg forward with knee straight about twelve to sixteen inches.
3. Turn toes inward—then keeping the knee straight and foot in, move the leg an equal distance to the rear.
4. Circle the leg outward (laterally) about twenty-four to thirty-six inches, then forward again.

Continue the motion ten to twelve repetitions, then reverse for another ten to twelve times. Repeat with opposite leg.

Keep the body erect and eyes forward. Try to make all movement from hip socket only. Concentrate on even circular motions, keeping knees straight and toes inward. Muscles in the hips often cramp from this even after weeks of conditioning. (Don't worry if yours do too!)

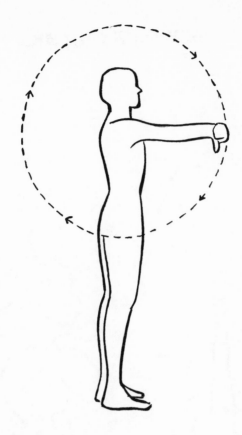

B. Arms

    1. Extend right arm forward.
    2. Turn thumb toward the ground.
    3. Raise arm overhead and swing through in a circle, keeping the elbow straight, ten to twelve repetitions.
    4. Reverse the motion, ten to twelve repetitions. Repeat with opposite arm.

Keep the body erect. Try to make movements smooth and flowing. The thumb position is important in that it puts the head of the humerus (upper arm) in its best alignment with the shoulder socket. (Same holds true for the toes in relation to the hip socket.) If pain (bursitis) occurs in the shoulder, slow down the speed and range of movement.

The arm and leg rotation exercises are given with the intent of loosening up the four ball and socket joints and major appendages. The advantage is in stimulating circulation and maintaining flexibility of these joints (*critical juncture* areas!)

V. KNEE BENDS ON TOES

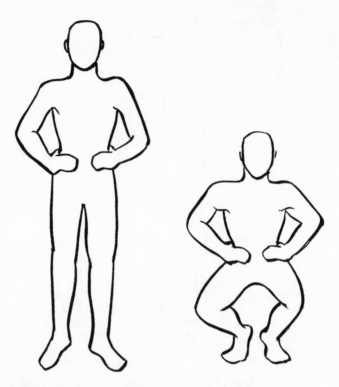

A. Begin with hands on the hips. For someone who has difficulty at first, place the hands further down the thigh for leverage. Stand with feet shoulder width apart, head up, back straight.
B. Exhale as you squat downward.
C. Inhale as you come up. Bounce slightly at the bottom before coming up. Concentrating on three counts—it's down on *one, two* with the bounce and up on *three*.
   Repeat seven times.

Keep eyes on a fixed spot for balance. This strengthens the knee and ankle ligaments, also the feet.

Modern myth: Knee bends are dangerous! Quite the contrary. Deep knee bends are not harmful to healthy knee joints. (Example: How many major league baseball catchers have their careers shortened because of knee problems?) However, *duck walking* can be harmful for some knee joints and lots of squats can slow down a sprinter's speed.

VI. "THE BARNYARD SHUFFLE" LOOSENER

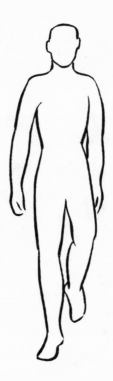

A. Stand on one foot. Bend forward at the waist.
B. Extend the opposite arm forward and the loose leg to the rear. Vigorously shake both hand and foot as if they had something on them that you wanted shaken off.
C. Reverse legs and repeat two to three times each.

This is an excellent loosener/relaxer. To be used repeatedly after knee bends or upon rising from seated or prone exercises. (Also establishes "Cross/Crawl" neurological balances.)

VII. HIP CIRCLE OR "HULA HOOP"

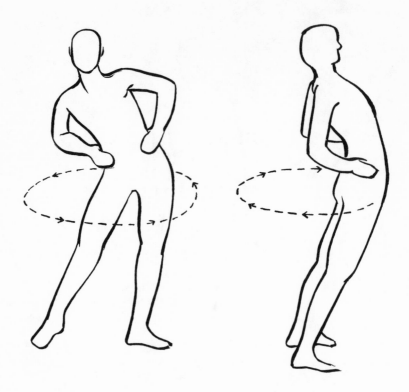

A. For the hip circle the feet are placed parallel, a bit wider than the shoulder width apart.

B. Bring hips well forward, clasp hands behind the back, then circle the hips, keeping the head and shoulders relatively stationary, trying to make a perfect circle. (It's as if you were standing in a barrel and trying to touch all sides as you go around.) This is to develop flexibility in the pelvic girdle and loosen up the lower back. Repeat seven times in each direction.

After the Hip Circles, repeat the Jangle, running in place. The effect here is to stir up the heartbeat again, stimulating circulation, and loosening the shoulder girdle by alternately reaching overhead with clenched fists.

VIII. FORWARD BENDS (Knees Bent)

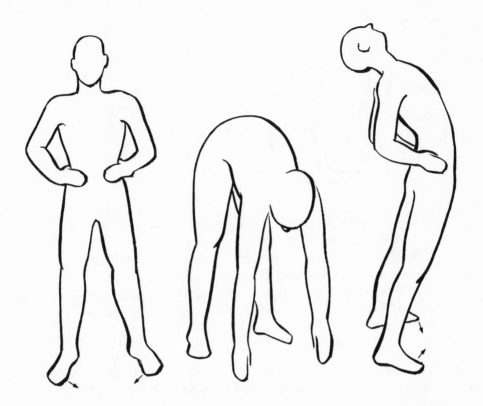

A. Place the feet wider than shoulder width apart with the toes pointed inward.
B. Bend forward at the waist, exhaling, bending as far as you can comfortably on *one,* then stretch further forward on *two, three* and *four.*
C. Raise up and stretch backward with the hands on the hips and then return. Repeat seven times.

Note: Pull the abdomen in tightly on *two, three* and *four* counts, exhaling further on each. Inhale deeply when coming erect. This is an excellent lymphatic pumping movement, and is also excellent for firming the lower abdomen.

IX. EGG ROLL

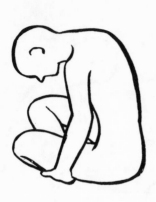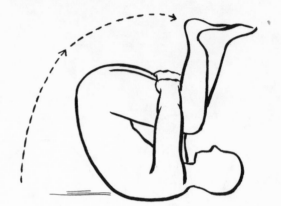

A. In a seated position grasp the hands behind the knees, crossing the feet if desired.
B. Keeping the chin down on the chest, raise the knees and roll back on the shoulders while exhaling.
C. Roll back and forth, up and down, on the spine, returning forward to the seated position each time. Repeat seven times.

This is excellent for keeping the spine flexible and properly aligned, as well as stimulating circulation in the internal organs. (Good to do at other times of the day as a single exercise.) Some floor padding is needed for comfortable Egg Rolls.

X. CERVICAL RELEASE (For Lymphatic Drainage)

This consists of pressure and massage to the 3rd cervical vertebra area.

A. While sitting, place thumb and forefinger together in back of neck, at the base of the skull.
B. Raise the chin, then press the fingertips firmly in the hollowmost spot, or so-called "nape" of the neck, near midline. This will be the area of the 3rd cervical. The 4th and 5th vertebrae just below, stick out prominently. Keep the pressure above them.
C. Lie back in a relaxed manner with knees up, chin raised, and continue the pressure two to four minutes, massaging any sore spots you may find there.

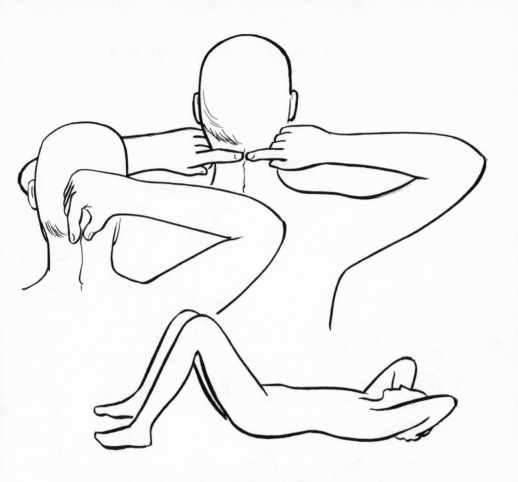

The lymphatic reflex technique is inserted at this point to promote lymph drainage throughout the major abdominal organs and especially in the eye, ear, nose and throat areas. *(It is also very helpful for alleviating headaches, sinus conditions, eye strain or fatigue from prolonged sitting at a desk, driving, etc!)*

Support the thumb and forefinger with the opposite hand, using the weight of head and shoulders for pressure. If you feel gurglings in the throat and abdomen, or popping of the ears and sinuses, these are signs of effectiveness. Be sure to keep the knees bent and the feet higher than the torso if possible. (A pillow or incline will help.) Keep the chin raised.

Caution: Do not maintain pressure for over four to five minutes, especially if you tend toward low blood pressure. Since this lymphatic release tends to lower blood pressure by relaxing normal nerve tension, do not get up quickly to resume any standing activity as this may result in temporary dizziness or difficulty in balance.

Note: Repeat the affirmation during the cervical release.

XI. ALTERNATE KNEE AND ELBOW TOUCH

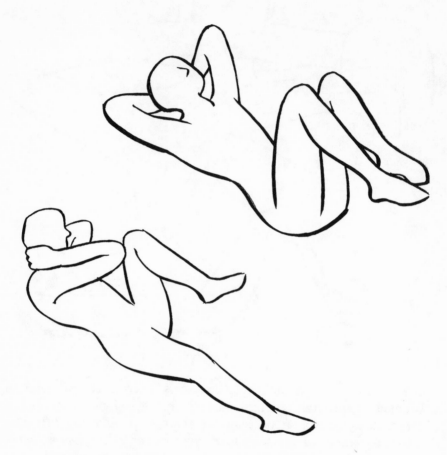

A. While still lying down, clasp hands behind the neck.
B. Raise the knees.
C. Alternately twist the torso, touching the elbows to the *inside* of the opposite knee. (The leg not being touched should extend straight out, toes pointed, slightly above the ground.)

    Repeat ten to twelve times.

Keep the chin down. Do not hold your breath, but breathe shallow throughout. This exercise strengthens the abdominal and groin muscles. Additionally, we use it here to place pressure on the abdomen in order to further promote lymphatic circulation and its return to the general venous circulation.

XII. SHOULDER STAND

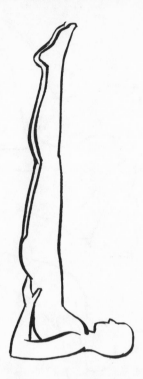

Do three more "Egg Rolls," then roll back to a shoulder stand, raising the legs to a vertical position, hands on sides for support. Hold position, breathing deeply, for fifteen to sixty seconds.

Caution: Do not attempt this if your neck is not in good condition, or if it has sustained past injuries. (However, some initial stiffness is normal as a result of these activities.) Also for individuals who are very stiff it might be better to wait three weeks, just doing the other exercises.

Try to elongate the neck. Keep the body straight. As an alternate, if shoulder stands are impractical, lie down with legs raised during this segment of the routine. (An incline board is most effective.) The shoulder stand is extremely important here in that it allows gravity to promote return circulation of the lymph to the subclavian veins—thus back into the general circulation—and on to the liver, kidneys, lungs and skin for excretion of waste substances.

Advanced students may prefer to spend more time with the shoulder stand, or add such movements as Leg Swings, the inverted Lotus, Plough, and return to Bridge position.

XIII. THE BRIDGE

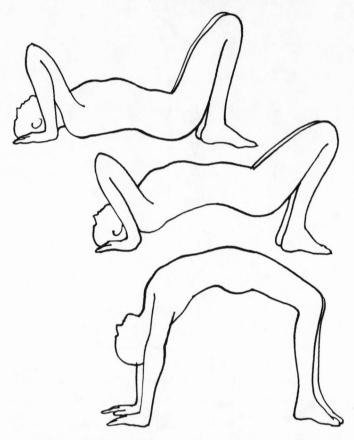

A. After returning to a supine position, pull the heels up close to the buttocks, arch the back, while pulling the neck in—then place hands palms down alongside the head.

B. Thrust the hips up with the back arched, push with hands so as to raise the shoulders until you are supporting the upper weight with hands and top of the head.

C. Breathe deeply, three to four breaths. Concentrate on getting as much arch into the lower back as possible.

D. Return to supine position. Relax, breathe deeply.

Advanced students may push up with arms extended into the "Wheel."

Caution: The bridge is a somewhat advanced pose for many, especially those who are in poor physical condition or getting along in years. Pace yourself accordingly.

XIV. THE FISH

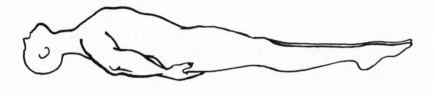

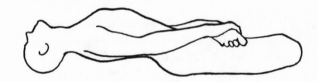

A. In supine position, place hands palms up under the buttocks, legs extended.
B. Raise to a half-seated position, supported by elbows.
C. Arch the back and elongate the neck, relaxing the head back as far as possible.
D. Breathe deeply through the nose, three to five repetitions.
E. Raise the head and slowly return to supine position. Relax, breathe deeply.
F. Repeat, with legs crossed or in a lotus position. When arched, try to get the head nearly back to floor level.

The advantages of the Fish are that it fills the upper lobes of the lungs more effectively than most any other exercise, at the same time adding stimulation and flexibility to the critical lymphatic junction areas of the upper chest and shoulders.

XV. LEG RAISES AND SIDE TORSION STRETCH

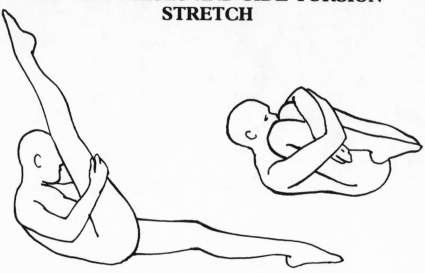

A. In supine position, elongate the right leg, toes pointed, then raise the leg, knee straight, while inhaling.
B. Grasp the leg (while holding the breath) and pull the knee firmly to the forehead. (Hold the position and the breath three to five seconds.)
C. Exhale while lowering the leg. Relax, take a deep breath.
D. Repeat with opposite leg. (Two to three repetitions for each leg).
E. Raise both legs together, again knees straight, inhaling. Pull in to forehead and hold.

For the Side Stretch:

A. At this point, exhale, bend the knees (knees together) and squeeze them tightly to the chest. Hold for several seconds.
B. Now drop the knees (still bent) to the right, extend the arms (spread eagled) and look left. Relax the abdomen, breathe deeply. (Relax further on exhaling.)
C. Reverse with knees to the left, looking right. Relax the midsection, breathe deeply. Relax further on exhaling.
D. Repeat, but instead of relaxing, stretch the left hip and shoulder away from each other as far as possible. Then breathe and relax. (See illustration for hooking ankle over knee for added stretch.)

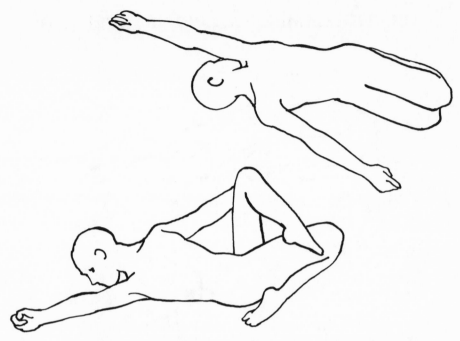

E. Reverse, stretching out the right hip and shoulder. Breathe and relax.

F. Return knees (still bent) to center. Again squeeze in to chest.

G. Straighten knees, pull in to forehead.

H. Lower legs to supine position. Relax, breathe deeply.

The order of breathing and relaxation is very important in the leg raises as well as in all subsequent exercises employing holding of the breath. By inhaling and holding the breath as the leg is pulled to the forehead, we effectively help force the spinal fluid down from the brain to the lowermost ends of the spinal cord (consequently a pumping effect). As we relax and breathe deeply we allow time for fresh blood to flow in with food, oxygen and fresh amounts of tissue fluid. The side stretch gives torsion and relaxation to the lower lumbar vertebrae and pelvic areas with little accompanying strain. This aids in preventing tendencies toward misalignment of the spinal vertebrae and sacro-lumbar joints—misalignments which can lead to reduced nerve and blood supply, or cause shooting pains, tenderness, muscle spasms, stiffness and soreness. (*Any exercise follower who experiences chronic pain and stiffness in the lower back, neck or shoulders should consult a chiropractic physician, osteopath or orthopedic physician for examination, x-rays, and/or professional opinion regarding the cause and correction of his condition.*)

XVI. THE CAMEL AND PELVIC STRETCH

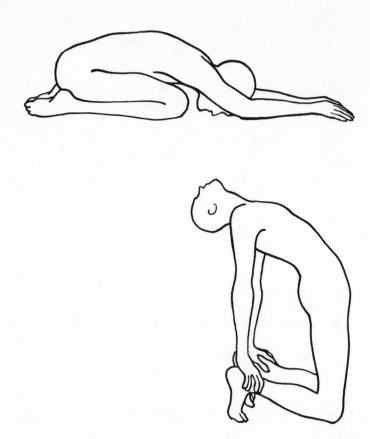

A. In a kneeling position sit back with legs apart so that feet and ankles are outside the hips.
B. Bow forward until the forehead touches the floor.
C. Grasp the ankles and pull the pelvis down as close to the floor as possible. Flatten the back and shoulders. Breathe deeply three to four breaths.
D. Raise up on knees and arch backward, head back as in the Fish.
E. Place hands on the heels then thrust the pelvis forward and up. Hold, breathing shallow, three to four breaths. Concentrate on arching the pelvis and low back. Repeat two to three repetitions.

XVII. SUPINE LAYOUT

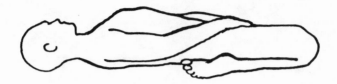

A. Begin from the Camel position as above, continuing from the previous exercise.
B. Raise up on knees, then lower the torso back until head and shoulders are flat on the floor. Hands are at sides or clasped across the abdomen, or clasping the feet.
C. Concentrate on relaxing the ankles and thigh muscles, plus getting the entire spine and abdomen as flat and straight as you can. (This may prove difficult for some at first. On the average, women are usually better than men on this one.) Hold for three to four breaths, then turn over and lie on the abdomen. Relax and loosen the feet, ankles and thighs.

This segment of Camel and Pelvic Stretch is very important in our progressive attempts to move the lymph. The camel position spreads the pelvis allowing the spinal fluid to flow more readily out from the lower brush ends of the spinal cord—at the same time contracting the muscles of the back and shoulders, thighs and buttocks, pumping lymph and venous blood away from these large muscle groups. On relaxation, abundant quantities of blood, with food and oxygen, flow into the muscles setting the stage for our next group of arching exercises, which are to be done in prone position. (Cobra, Locust, Boat and Bow.) *Note:* Breathing and relaxation during these exercises is on the same principle that we concentrated upon during leg raises. Between each exercise place the hands to the sides, head to one side and relax completely, breathing as deeply as possible.

XVIII. THE COBRA

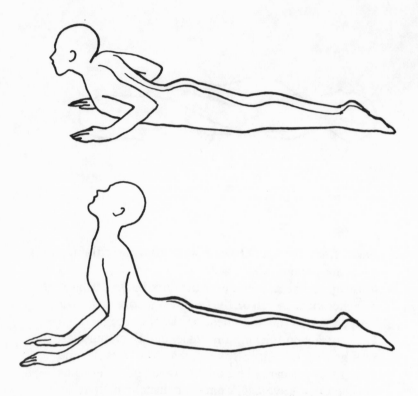

A. In prone position, place hands at shoulder level, raise up (inhaling) arching the back and neck as far as possible before applying pressure with the hands.

B. Hold the breath, press up till the elbows are straightened.

C. Relax the lower back. Hold until there is need for air.

D. Return slowly to the prone position, exhaling as you do.

E. Relax, take a deep breath or two.

    Repeat two to three repetitions.

Concentrate on an even flow of movement, breathing and relaxation. Keep eyes closed for better concentration. Advancing students may wish to include the Swan. This is done in the raised Cobra position by bending the knees and bringing the feet up together close to the head, then turning the head right and left, attempting to touch the head and feet.

XIX. THE LOCUST

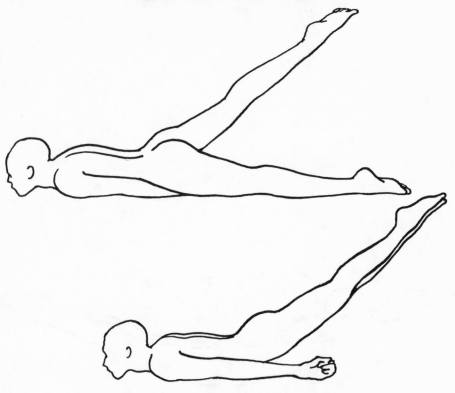

A. In prone position, clench fists and place the hands, palms up, under the upper thighs.

B. Raise the head slightly to where the chin rests lightly on the floor. (It should stay in this position throughout, while the legs are being raised and lowered.)

C. Stretch out the right leg, pointing the toes and elongating. Then, inhaling, raise the leg, knee straight, as high as possible. Keep the hips level. The thigh should come up high off the fist. The hip should stay down as much as possible.

D. Hold the breath and the pose until air is needed, then lower the leg, exhaling. Relax and take a deep breath or two.

E. Repeat with alternate leg, two to three repetitions each.

As students advance they will no doubt include the full locust, raising both feet simultaneously. For greater height on the full locust turn the hands palms down with fingers extended.

XX. THE BOAT

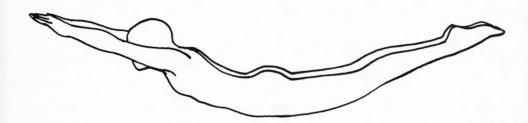

A. In prone position, extend the arms overhead. Stretch
   out and elongate arms and legs to their fullest extension.
B. Inhale, arching the back, raising the head, arms and
   legs.
C. Hold the breath, concentrating on keeping everything
   up—chin up, eyes up, fingertips up, toes up. Hold
   without straining unduly.
D. Exhale, lower and relax. Breathe deeply.
   Repeat two to three repetitions.

XXI. THE BOW

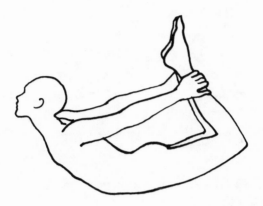

A. In prone position, bend the knees, grasp the ankles and pull them up close to the buttocks.
B. Inhaling, raise the head and arch the back, pressing the ankles away from the body. (Try to bring the thighs up off the floor as the feet press away from the hands.)
C. Hold the breath and tension, keeping the shoulders back as far as possible until air is needed. Again, hold without straining.
D. Exhale, lower and relax. Breathe deeply.
    Repeat two to three repetitions.

An advanced movement is to rock forward and backward on the abdomen while in a bowed position. (Excellent for strengthening abdominal muscles.)

Rocking is activated simply by moving the chin down and forward, or back as desired. Shallow breathing is recommended if you care to rock for very long.

XXII. YOGA MUDRA

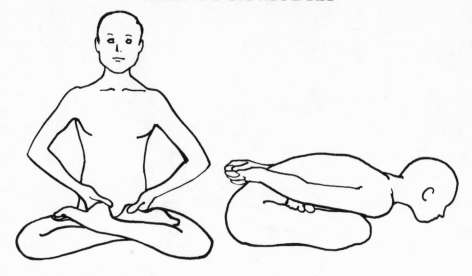

A. Assume a cross-legged seated position. (Lotus for advanced students.)
B. Bend forward, exhaling, as far as possible. (Arms may be extended forward or clasped behind the back or neck as preferred.)
C. Hold the pose, concentrating on relaxing and extending the lower back. (Upper back should be relatively straight.)
D. Breathe shallow and with each exhalation further relax the lower back in this manner:
   1. Breathe out "all weariness."
   2. Breathe out "all tensions."
   3. Breathe out "all inflexibility."
   4. Breathe out "all negativity."
   5. Breathe out "all hostility."
   6. Breathe out "all of the past"
      (negative Karma.)
E. Raise up with the eyes closed, (Yoga Mudra).
   1. Breathe in "peace."
   2. Breathe in "strength."
   3. Breathe in "vitality."

The Yoga Mudra is an excellent mental/emotional exercise in addition to its specific advantage of increasing flexibility. An obvious "lift" will be felt as one rises out of the forward position. Include Bellows Breathing here, twenty to forty repetitions.

XXIII. SHOULDER LOOSENER AND "BALINESE DANCER" MOVEMENT

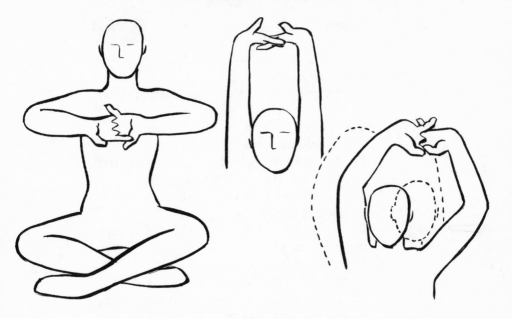

A. In seated position, clasp hands in front then turn palms down and away from the body.

B. Raise arms overhead and stretch, bringing the shoulders up high behind the ears. Raise and lower the shoulders to the ears, rapidly, ten to twelve times.

C. With the hands still overhead, relax the shoulders and sway the head side-to-side in the manner of the Balinese Dancers. Face straight to the front, jaw maintained level throughout. Repeat ten to twelve times.

D. Move the head forward and back, three to four times. Then in a circle, three to four times in each direction.

E. Stretch overhead, then relax. Extend the arms out and shake them to loosen hands, arms and shoulders.

The head should move as a pendulum, ears slightly forward of the shoulders. Move the shoulders. Movement should center mostly in the upper shoulder area. (Practice in front of a mirror.) An eye exercise can be added here by focusing the vision away from the direction of movement.

This combination brings both strength and flexibility to the neck and shoulders while stimulating circulation and toning the skin (good for avoiding or reducing double chins!).

XXIV. FACE AND SCALP MASSAGE

A. Rub the palms together vigorously until the hands become quite warm, then cup them over the eyes. (Concentrate on relaxing the eyeballs as the warmth penetrates—feel them melt.)

B. When the warmth is dissipated begin massaging with fingertips in this order:
   1. Upper lids, outward over the temples.
   2. Lower lids, outward over the temples.
   3. Brush the upper lids downward in butterfly wing fashion. (Observe the patterns of light.)
   4. The temples in a circular motion.
   5. In front of the ears.
   6. Behind and below the ears. (Tug and squeeze the ear lobes.)
   7. Down the side of the neck.
   8. Gently about the throat and Adam's Apple.
   9. Under the jaw (using the tops of the fingers).
   10. Lower gums and jaw muscles.
   11. Upper gums.
   12. Cheekbones.
   13. Nose.
   14. Bridge of the nose (important area).
   15. Brows.
   16. Forehead.
   17. Scalp.
   18. Back and sides of scalp.
   19. Base of skull (occipital areas).
   20. Base of skull, behind and below the ears (mastoid area).
   21. Muscles in back of the neck (raise chin).
   22. Vigorously rub the entire scalp with fingers and palms or knuckles, then "gather up all negativity" and literally "throw it away." Finally, slap hands together, flick the fingertips outward, and rub them on the ground.

The facial massage not only moves the lymph along and firms the tissues, it also stimulates numerous reflex points in both face and scalp. Normally each of the areas noted for massage will only require a few moments attention, however, when some soreness or sensitivity is experienced it would be well to return to these areas later for additional treatment.

Note: Anyone adding eye exercise to their program is advised to follow such exercises with facial massage as prescribed here. Also if the eyes are being worked on without previous general warm-up exercises it would be well to precede them with a few Egg Rolls and the Cervical Release for assisting lymphatic drainage.

XXV. ELBOW SQUEEZE

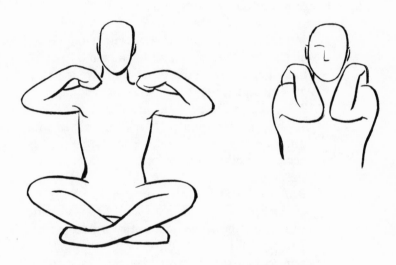

A. Place the finger tips on the shoulders and bring the elbows and forearms tightly together, then inhale deeply. Hold for a count of three; chin pressed tightly to chest.

B. With finger tips still on the shoulders bring the elbows back as far as possible, exhale and hold tightly for three counts. Repeat three to four times. Relax, shaking and loosening the arms and shoulders.

Keep the elbows on the same level throughout. This is essentially an isometric exercise which strengthens the pectoral regions and also stimulates the lymphatic circulation throughout the bust and shoulder areas (excellent for firming the bustline). The inhalation stimulates the thyroid and main lymphatic junction areas.

XXVI. CHEST AND SHOULDER MASSAGE

A. Place tips of the thumbs at the juncture of upper arms and pectorals.
B. Massage with thumb pads (and sides of forefingers) in the outer pectoral regions, concentrating on any sore spots.
C. Continue inward under the collar bones.
D. With the fingertips at the center of the chest, proceed downward along the breastbone massaging between the ribs with the fingertips. Again, concentrate on any sore spots.
E. Massage under the ribs out to the sides.
F. Taking one side at a time:
   1. Massage up the side with opposite hand. Grasp all the flesh possible under the arm and the back including the shoulder blade, and give it a good general squeezing, rubbing and kneading.
   2. Take the entire pectoral muscle in hand and apply pressure toward the ribcage along with some circular movement. (Some females may need to modify this according to their breast size.)
   3. Roll the flesh under the upper arm with the top of the opposite hand; then with hand pressure and kneading, work on the entire arm from forearm up, squeezing the forearm, elbow, upper arm and finally the shoulder cap. As with the facial massage, these areas contain many lymphatic reflex points which should receive additional attention if they are found to be extra sensitive. Female participants will find this to be an appropriate time for breast examination, to ascertain the presence of any unusual tenderness, lumps, swollen lymph nodes, etc. Obviously any suspicious conditions should be presented to an appropriate physician.

Extreme Caution: Under certain infectious conditions massage can prove harmful—by spreading disease germs, toxins or even cancerous cells which would be better kept localized.

Do not massage any areas where there are abnormally swollen glands, pimples, boils or infections. Also, do not undergo general or specific body massage anytime there is an elevated temperature or inflammation present in the body (thus a suspected infection) without the cognizant approval of a physician. The cautions noted here also hold true for vigorous exercise or physical activity which might spread infections and aggravate some conditions, thus overriding any advantages that might be gained from such activity.

A very important general note on massage: Since massage affects the venous blood vessels as well as the lymphatic circulation, note that most of these vessels have valves to prevent backward movement of blood and lymphatic fluids. Any strong reverse massage or pressure can injure the valves and the vessels themselves. (Varicose veins are a classic example of such a breakdown from reverse pressures.) *Massage should always be directed away from the extremities and toward the heart.* Massage of the torso (back, chest and abdomen) should be directed inward and upward, or toward the spine. Massage of varicose vein areas should be avoided by anyone other than professionally qualified therapists.

Now that we have effectively concentrated on loosening the shoulder girdle we are ready to move on to an equally important area—the pelvic girdle. (The pelvic chakras are often considered to be the "Seat of the Soul" and deserving of special attention.)

XXVII. GROIN AND PELVIC CONDITIONING (PLUS FOOT MASSAGE)

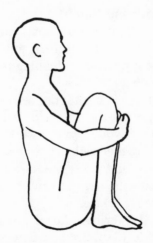

A. "Straight Arrow"
   1. In seated position bend the knees (close together) up to the chest.

2. Clasp arms about the knees and exhale, squeezing them close to the body.
3. Inhale, straightening up as erect as possible, elongating the entire spine, flattening the back, raising the head and shoulders so as to be as tall as you can be while seated. (Pull the belly in at the same time.) Hold for ten to twenty seconds.

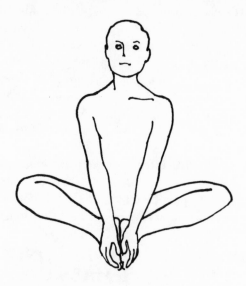

B. Buttocks Rock and Butterfly
1. Drop the knees wide apart and placing the bottoms of the feet together, pull the heels in close to the groin (hands holding the feet in position throughout).
2. Sit up straight, pull the belly in, then rock side to side on the buttocks ten to twelve times (longer if you need the work on this area).
3. Keeping the head and the spine erect and heels in, raise and lower the knees in butterfly wing movements, ten to twelve times (as low as you can move them).
4. Stop. Lower both knees as close to the floor as possible. (Advanced students will have achieved a straight right angle degree of flexibility.)

C. Forward Bend in Butterfly Position
1. With feet still hand held close to the groin, in-

hale deeply, then bend forward, exhaling, bringing the forehead as close to the feet as possible.

2. Breathe shallow and concentrate on relaxation of the lower back and groin muscles (in same fashion as in the Yoga Mudra). Advanced students will bring their foreheads completely to the feet while keeping the spine as straight as possible.
3. Raise up with eyes closed as in the Yoga Mudra.
4. Breathe in "Peace."
   Breathe in "Joy."
   Breathe in "Tranquility."
5. Extend the legs. Loosen the feet, ankles and legs, rolling them side to side.

D. Foot Massage
   1. Still seated, inhaling, bring one foot up to rest on the opposite thigh. Loosen the hips and thigh by pressing the knee down and up as in the Butterfly.
   2. Massage as follows:
      a. Spread the longitudinal arch, pulling apart with both hands.
      b. Pull on the toes (all of them at once).
      c. Squeeze the lower part of the foot, firmly applying torsion first in one direction then the other.
      d. Massage the bottom of the foot firmly with the palm and heel of the opposite hand. (Again, make a note of sensitive reflex areas for further attention.)
      e. Massage the toes individually, using thumbs and forefingers. Squeeze and rotate the toe tips as you would in playing with marbles.
      f. Massage the top of the foot with fingertips, making movements away from the toes and between the metatarsal bones.
      g. Next, massage the entire ankle area, using both hands, fingers and palms, apply special attention to the juncture of heel and achilles tendon.
      h. Now move up the calf alternately squeezing,

rotating, and rubbing. (The calf muscles should be consciously relaxed.)

i. Finally, give attention to the outer muscles lying alongside the shinbone (Tibialas Anterior).

j. Again massage the bottom—toes, foot and heel—using a vigorous knuckle rub.

E. Leg and Groin Loosening

1. Cradle the leg, bringing the bent knee out to the side, the heel close in to the crotch.

2. Swing the knee out horizontally to the side as far as possible, then back in, seven times.

3. With the foot close to the crotch, circle the foot (holding it with both hands), seven times in each direction.

4. Squeeze the knee in under the chin, then grasp the foot with both hands and raise it as follows:

   a. Toes to chin.

   b. Toes to nose.

   c. Toes to forehead.

   d. Heel to the Pineal (bottom of foot atop the head). (Advanced students will bring the foot up behind the head.)

5. Grasp the outside of the foot with one hand same side hand as foot) straighten the knee out as far as possible and wave the leg out to the side and back seven times. (Keep the back straight as you do.)

6. Flex the knee, bringing the leg down, around, and under the buttocks (opposite leg forward and straight). Sit directly on the foot (toes to rear) with the heel/ankle bone intruding into one's anal areas. Bend forward exhaling and stroke the extended leg (much as a harpist would) four times. (Don't actually touch the leg.) On the last stroke raise up with both arms extending (as an unfolding lotus blossom). Let one's vibrations flow freely upward in the process.

Repeat foot massage, leg and groin looseners with the opposite leg.

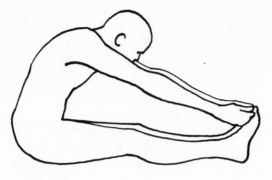

F. Forward Bend
1. Assume a seated position with legs extended, knees close together.
2. Raise the arms overhead, inhaling.
3. Bend forward at the waist, exhaling, stretching as far as possible.
4. Grasp either the legs, ankles, or feet according to your degree of flexibility. Hold the pose, breathing shallow, concentrating on relaxing the lower back and hamstring muscles.
5. Raise up, stretching and inhaling. Repeat two to three times. (Then roll the legs side to side, to loosen and relax.)

Bring upper body well forward and pull the belly in before finally bending as far as possible. Advanced students will attain the ideal position of chest and forehead resting fully on the legs with knees and back held straight.

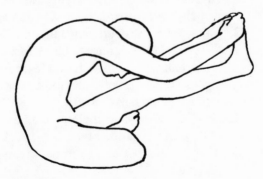

G. Groin Stretch
1. In seated position with legs extended, bend one knee up and out, placing the bottom of the foot on the inside of the opposite thigh. Pull the heel up high into the crotch.

2. Raise the arms overhead, inhaling and bend over the extended leg, exhaling and stretching. Same technique as in the Forward Bend. Repeat with opposite leg, two to three repetitions each side.

Note: The upper body position can vary on this in two basic ways: (1) With shoulders level, the face comes down directly on the knee. (2) With shoulders turned, the upper body performs a side bend bringing the side of the face down to leg level. The latter variation is more difficult, thus more advanced. We suggest that both be considered and worked on.

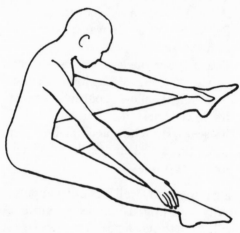

H. Straddle Bend

1. In seated position, extend the legs (knees straight) wide apart, as far as you can.
2. Raise the arms overhead, inhaling.
3. Keeping knees straight, bend forward at the waist, exhaling. Grasp the ankles or feet according to your degree of flexibility (or arms may extend straight overhead).
4. Hold the pose as in the forward bend, concentrating on relaxation of the lower back and hamstrings. (Keep the upper back as straight as possible.)
5. Raise up, stretch and repeat two to three times.

Note: An advanced variation of the straddle position is to grasp the feet while seated, then raise the feet high in the air while straightening out the knees. (The trick is in maintaining one's balance.)

I. Yoga Mudra (See XXII, Page   )

This is a repeat—partly as a final forward stretch, partly to show how the lower back and groin muscles have become more flexible and relaxed as a result of the stretching and loosening activities. (I often refer to this as an "Instant Karma" exercise, noting that some Karma can be very pleasant.)

Raise up from the Yoga Mudra, this time:
—Breathing in "Peace."
—Breathing in "Joy."
—Breathing in "Tranquility."

(At this point I usually feel so peaceful and tranquil that I don't want to continue exercising—but there are more worthwhile things to come!

So before moving on I usually take time here to include a healing affirmation, one that is in our attitudes and emotions book. You may find it worth adding here too.)

"Father/Mother God, with Thy Grace, I will the life force to flow, through each cell of my being—throughout this entire day—healing, regenerating, this entire form and spirit."

Also at this point I find a short period of "Bellows Breathing" is helpful. As with the affirmations this is optional for anyone following the entire routine.

J. Bellows Breathing
1. Still seated, with eyes closed, breathe deeply in and out through the nose, concentrating on ballooning the belly outward on inhalation and contracting it tightly on exhalation.
2. After a few preliminary breaths, contract and relax the lower abdomen as quickly and forcefully as you can. (The breath will move in and out the nose without the customary aid of chest muscles.) Continue until the abdominal muscles call out for rest.)

Do not try to inhale. Concentrate on the abdomen and keep the chest uninvolved.

Note: An advanced variation of the Bellows is attained by concentrating on the diaphram muscle and making it force inhalation and exhalation in a more rapid sequence, much like a panting dog. (This requires close coordination between the diaphragm and abdominal muscles.)

Now we are ready for our final segment of exercises (which we begin in standing position). On rising you will find that the legs feel somewhat heavy and unwilling to move very rapidly. This is partly because of the workout we've given them, partly because we have not had our circulation speeded up for a while. For this reason it is important to "jangle" vigorously and get good heart/lung acceleration before our closing exercises—which concentrate on a thorough recycling of the lymphatic circulation through the tissues of the body. (A forward stretch with knee clasp is a good practical addition here before jangling; also, "The Barnyard Shuffle.")

XXVIII. JANGLE (Palms Up)

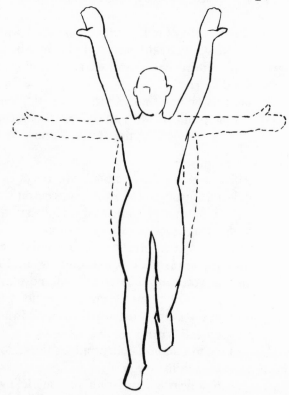

A. While running in place and getting well loosened up, take three deep breaths (again, always inhaling through the nose.)

B. Still running, slowly raise the hands, palms up, over-head and stretch high up, inhaling as you do. (Very important! Concentrate on this movement.)
C. Lower the hands, palms down, bringing them to the side and rear. Repeat five to seven repetitions.

This variation of arm movements while running in place loosens the shoulders and raises the rib cage more forcibly than when we raise just one arm at a time. Again we are concentrating on the critical lymphatic junctures in the upper chest and shoulder areas.

Note: The palms up position is extremely important here. (Try it in other ways and feel the difference.)

XXIX. FLAT FOOTED SQUATS

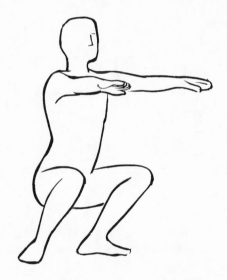

A. Place the feet shoulder-width apart, toes pointed out-ward about thirty degrees.
B. Squat, forcibly, exhaling as you do, keeping the heels flat on the ground, extending the arms straight for-ward for balance. (Keep the head up and back straight.) Hold in the "down" position, fully exhaling before coming erect. While there, forcibly contract the lower abdominal muscles (fine lymphatic pumping movement).
C. Come erect, inhaling deeply—chest high, shoulders back, fists on hips. Repeat five to seven repetitions.

If this proves difficult at first, do it between a pair of chair tops for assistance. (A stall bar or exercise bar can be used in the same manner.) This is one of the very best exercises for strengthening and firming the upper thighs, buttocks and lower abdomen. Should you desire to lose inches off these areas, the repetitions should be raised to fifty to two hundred per day (in sets of twenty to twenty-five). A variation of hand/arm position is to place the palms together close to the chest in prayer position as you squat. This is more comfortable to some than the extended position.

XXX. KNEE AND GROIN STRENGTHENER

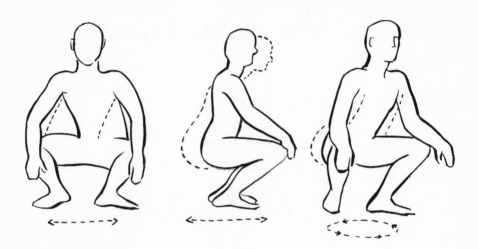

A. While still in the squat position, bring the elbows inside the knees and rock side to side, coming up on the toes, four repetitions.
B. Then rock forward and back four times.
C. Circle right, then left, four complete circles, keeping the lower abdominal muscles pulled in tight and hips low as you do.

This may prove difficult at first, but once mastered will keep the ankles, knees, groin and pelvic areas in excellent condition.

This will not adversely affect anyone who has healthy knee joints. If you've had injuries in these areas, be careful. If balance is a problem concentrate your awareness on the tips of your toes (even though you may not be seeing them). Also, the arm position can be varied by clasping hands or elbows. This, too, may aid in better balance.

XXXI. THE CROW

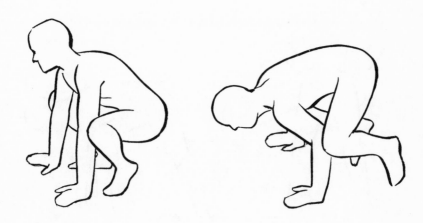

A. Still in the squat position with elbows inside the knees, place the palms flat on the ground.
B. With the knees supported by the elbows, slowly rock forward until the body is entirely supported by the hands.
C. Hold position for up to a count of seven (longer if desired).

If at first your arms cannot support your weight, practice rocking forward, putting only as much weight on the hands and elbows as you can hold. This is essentially an isometric exercise. It strengthens the hands, wrists, forearms and shoulders, while developing balance and mental discipline. Also it is recommended as a good preparation exercise for those who wish to advance to doing Handstands, the Scorpion or Peacock.

XXXII. ALTERNATE SIDE BEND AND TOE TOUCH

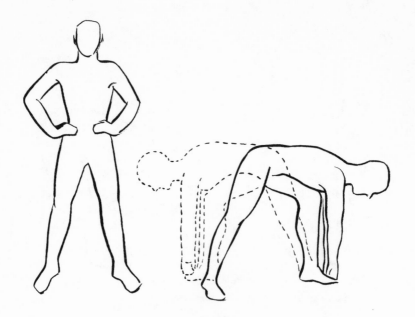

A. Stand with feet well apart, toes pointed outward.

B. Bend to one side, exhaling at the same time. Bend the knee on that side while keeping the opposite knee straight. (Keep the shoulders level to the ground.)

C. Touch (and touch a second time) the outside of the foot with both hands, while depressing the ribs upon the thigh.

D. Come erect, then turn and repeat to the opposite side. Repeat four to seven repetitions to each side.

Be sure to press the ribs down firmly on the thigh. (You may find that grasping the ankles helps.) This stimulates the liver and gall bladder on the right side, the spleen and pancreas on the left. *Breathe deeply throughout!* Excellent for firming and trimming the thighs, buttocks and waistline. It also strengthens the sacroiliac ligaments and attachments without putting undue strain on the lower back (again, another fine lymphatic pumping movement).

XXXIII. TIGER STRETCH (WITH VACUUM AND BUTTOCKS TIGHTENER)

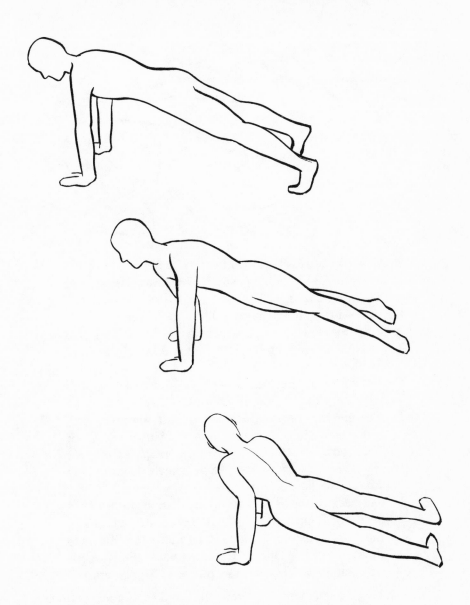

A. Begin from a pushup position, then sag at the waist (elbows straight, knees just off the ground), twisting the pelvis side to side (three to four times) to loosen the lower back.

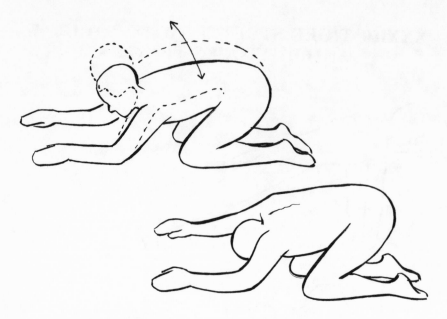

B. Drop the knees (keeping elbows straight and chin up) to the arched or Cobra position. The lower back should be fully relaxed.

C. Flex—bringing the buttocks back to the heels—exhaling, head down. Sway side to side four repetitions. (Do this as a loosener on both the first and last of the Tiger Stretches.)

D. Rock forward, extending the knees, again to the Cobra position, inhaling as you do.

E. Keeping the knees and elbows straight, lower the head and exhale while raising the hips to an inverted "V" or "up" position. *Hold for three deep breaths keeping the jaw and neck very relaxed.* (Bring heels down to help stretch the hamstrings.)

F. Sag back to the arched position, then again to flexed position. Repeat four to seven repetitions, ending in the "up" position and holding there for fifteen to thirty seconds. (During the last two to three repetitions, add the Vacuum and Buttocks Tighteners.)

Make the movements flow gracefully and rhythmically. Breathe and stretch deliberately as fully as possible.

Important Note: Combined with the Abdominal Vacuum and Buttocks Tightener (which follow) this is the very best single exercise of the entire routine. Or, if you were to do only one exercise each day this would be the one to practice faithfully.

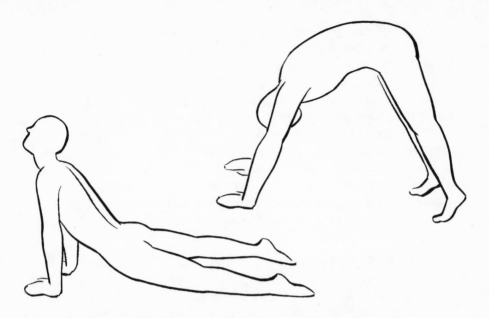

Elements of several Edgar Cayce recommendations are combined in the Tiger Stretch. These were given for all manner of lower circulatory problems—edema, varicose veins, hemorrhoids, prostate or uterine problems, constipation, etc.

The Tiger Stretch is especially recommended for females at the onset of their menstrual periods. (At such times do more repetitions and hold longer in the flexed position. Repeat twice a day for fifteen to thirty minutes or until discomfort passes.)

A. Vacuum (Abdominal Lift) (To be added during the Flexed position in the Tiger Stretch.)
   1. After two or three preliminary deep breaths, forcibly exhale as much air as possible.
   2. Consciously keep the nose and throat closed and raise the diaphragm as if inhaling—attempting to pull the internal organs up to the spine. (Do not take air in, however.)
   3. Hold this for several seconds until the need for air is apparent, then relax, take two to four deep breaths and repeat.

Repeat the vacuum repetitions during each of the last two to four Tiger Stretches.

Concentrate on lifting (and at the same time contracting) all the inner muscles, beginning from the heels and moving upward along the spine (including even the eyeballs; also, the anal sphincter and genital areas).

The flexed position brings the internal organs into their proper locations and alignment. The lift not only aids in tightening the mesenteries (connective tissue sheaths which help keep the organs in place) but also pulls the lymph out of the mesenteries/lacteals and internal organs. During the relaxed breathing period, fresh blood with food and oxygen flows more readily into these areas.

Advanced students may also practice this in the vertical position—using an in and out movement much like a reverse of the Bellows Breathing. Also, by pushing down with hands on knees the abdominal muscles will isolate and stand out (called The Rope). Masters of the Rope can make it move readily in and out or side to side with rolling motions by proper pressure and muscle control. (It's very good for the abdomen.)

B. Buttocks Tightener (to be done with The Vacuum).
   1. After the Abdominal Vacuum, move to the Arched or Cobra position.
   2. With chin raised, elbows and knees straight, forcibly contract the muscles of the buttocks and lower back. Inhale, pushing up with the head back.
   3. Hold tightly, three to four counts, then relax, drop the head and exhale deeply. Repeat three times during each of the Tiger Stretches which include the Vacuum. (It is well to include The Lion here too—with tongue fully extended downward, eyes forced up.)
   4. Move to the "Up" position, take three deep breaths and continue with the Tiger Stretch.

Note: This effectively ties in with the Abdominal Vacuum in promoting lymphatic circulation. It will also help firm the buttocks and strengthen the groin muscles. Additionally it is well recommended for individuals with hemorrhoid problems. (Do this regularly and you'll probably never have them!)

Moving into the "Up" (inverted) position allows the lymph to flow more readily into the subclavian veins and rushes large quantities of blood through the head. Advanced students will find seven full Tiger Stretches to be an excellent number—with the Vacuum and Buttocks Tightener included during the last four.

So ends the Daily Dozen exercise routine. A period of meditation afterwards is also extremely beneficial. (And highly recommended!)

6 Cautionary Thoughts and Health Tips

One can scarcely do any exercise that does not have its counterpart in Yoga. This in itself creates a problem for any practitioner of Yoga. One cannot begin to practice all the Yoga exercises or Asanas that are available, so some selectivity must be made. (This is why we suggest the Daily Dozen routine be followed initially.)

Unless the newcomer has a competent teacher or a strong background in health and physical education, plus knowledge of anatomy, physiology and kinesiology, he or she is very unlikely to select a suitable variety of exercises and put them in proper continuity. (Again, the Daily Dozen provides an ideal selection.)

An unfortunately small percentage of the Yoga teachers I've observed (at well known Yoga centers and elsewhere), have a good knowledge of body mechanics and physiology. (And I've never heard any one of them mention lymphatic circulation.) Also, most Yoga teachers, and Yoga books pay little attention to getting the circulation elevated at times such as we do in the Daily Dozen. I feel that heart/lung capacity should be considered and worked on by everyone after they have properly conditioned themselves through the first twelve-week period of the Daily Dozen. Jogging, swimming and cycling are excellent in this respect. (I believe a majority of individuals not exercising regularly before this will need six months to perfect the program. Dr. Shealy.)

Headstands Definitely Are Not For Everyone. Too many older people experience cervical vertebra problems when attempting them. I don't recommend headstands (or The Plough) for anyone, at least until after an initial twelve weeks of conditioning, and then only if the individual is not overweight and has never had any neck injuries. Also during initial attempts there should be an instructor present to aid in "spotting" to avoid abrupt falls. Not for beginners, period!

The Seated "Spinal Twist" Also Is Not For Everyone. Some individuals with spinal curvatures or misalignments can do themselves more harm than good with this pose. (The side stretch while lying down is gentle and easy on the spine.)

Prolonged Forced Breathing. This should not be attempted until a person is in excellent physical/emotional condition.

In general, however, it is better to perform a poor selection of Yoga exercises in an unfavorable continuity rather than not doing anything at all.

Jogging. Is also not for everyone. (It is especially bad for those over fifty-five who wish to start to condition themselves in this manner, according to Dr. C. Norman Shealy.) I agree. Anyone with foot problems, spinal curvatures, hip socket or spinal disc problems may aggravate them by attempting to join the jogging fad. Also, joggers tend to develop rigid and inflexible bodies unless they either practice Yoga or do regular stretching exercises along with jogging. In general, jogging is excellent for developing heart/lung competency and physical stamina. At the same time, anyone "past twenty-nine" who takes up the sport should first have a medical check-up, especially if he has been doing no running for a long time. Consider Power Walking (below) in lieu of Jogging.

Walking and Hiking. The more the better, especially in natural surroundings with plenty of fresh air. A daily walk is recommended for all.

Power Walking. An excellent stimulator/conditioner has been promoted by former "Mr. Universe" Steve Reeves. "Power Walking" entails walking in full vigorous strides with arms swinging forcibly to shoulder level. Breathing is done on count with full forced staccato inhalations/exhalations, three to five counts for each. Work up to twenty or thirty minutes a day, walking as fast as conditioning permits. Lengthen strides as far as attainable.

Note: Footwear should be comparable as for jogging. Both best done on grass or soft surfaces. (Concentrating on the breathing counts becomes an effective form of meditation.)

Isometrics. Like jogging, isometrics tend to reduce flexibility if not interspersed with a good bit of stretching and loosening of joints, muscles and tendons. Actually a good bit of yoga is isometric in nature. I prefer (and recommend) a balance of both isometric (stationary tension or pressures) and isotonic (moving tension) activities. (The Daily Dozen provides both in abundance.)

Weight Training. Hardly anyone appreciates weightlifters or body builders other than other weightlifters and bodybuilders. I'm favorably prejudiced since I did do a fair amount of weight training in my teens and early twenties. In general it is excellent for teenagers and athletes using weight training in conjunction with other sports where more strength is desired. Heavy lifting is hard on the low back though, so most people are better off using reasonably comfortable poundages for most exercises. A good way to keep strong and fit, but again there is a need to work additionally on flexibility and heart/lung competency.

Swimming. Unless we have access to a pool, lake or ocean, most of us do only an occasional bit of real swimming. One of the very best all around conditioners if you have the water, skill and persistence to work at it. The same holds true for surfing. (Especially good for lymphatic movement because of zero gravity effect.)

Cycling. What has emerged more or less as a fad in recent years will become even more of a movement what with our projected energy/fuel cost problems. Good exercise, but again its adherents need to stretch out those tightened hamstrings and hunched over shoulders that result from long rides. Also proper adjustment of seat is essential.

Golf. Once described by Mark Twain as "A good walk spoiled," golf is a relatively expensive and time consuming activity if only exercise is desired. Great for celebrities, professionals, spectators and those so inclined.

Commercial Health Clubs & Spas. The problem with many of these is that they are operated by salesmen rather than educators, with life memberships more in mind than their patron's physical well-being. Good places to exercise if you don't mind spending the money to do it.

Skiing. Not for the over twenty-nine crowd unless you've been doing it all your life. Exhilarating sport and good exercise, but sad to say, almost everyone eventually ends up in a cast somewhere along the way.

Tennis. A good conditioner as long as the elbows and shoulders hold up. The same holds true for Squash and Paddleball. Should be taken up only after three to six months of general conditioning.

Handball. Excellent for conditioning and co-ordination, especially the four-wall variety. (My own personal all-time favorite athletic activity.) Also squash, paddleball and racquetball.

Volley Ball. Excellent invigorating game for groups of all ages. Not one that of itself will develop much strength or endurance however. (Unless played in the sand!)

Bowling. About the same could be said as for volleyball, though bowling is even less advantageous for all around coordination and activity.

Baseball, Basketball, Football, Soccer. Fine spectator sports for our over twenty-nine group. Participation is not recommended unless you've continued straight on through from youth.

Horseback Riding. This has always impressed me as being excellent exercise for the horse. A good way to get around in rough country if you have a steed, but I've never seen a rider or a cowboy appear to be very loose jointed or flexible upon dismounting. Fine if you like horses.

Sailing, Rowing, Canoeing. These are all excellent, though again they are unlikely to be used as a consistent daily form of exercise.

Folk Dancing. Good, stimulating exercise, plus fun for the participants. However, few people dance often enough to keep in condition by this alone. Disco dancing is equally stimulating.

Gardening. Stretching, flexing, bending, kneeling, and squatting. The average gardener can stay in excellent condition. (This holds true for housework and general cleaning too.) However, if not in good condition, it's a potential way of injuring the back and other body parts.

Stretching, Flexing and Flicking. Hardly anyone does enough of this in routine living. We highly recommend it as a way of life for everyone! (Again, consider the animals—cats, dogs, horses, etc.—and how they stretch, shake, yawn and relax.) Emphasis on stretching and flexibility has lately "arrived" in athletic circles, such as among professional football players. Naturally, the flexible well-stretched-out athlete is less inclined to experience injuries, muscle tears, etc.

It is well to learn muscle control or "flicking." By systematically flexing and shaking, flicking, and/or massaging muscle groups, the lymph is moved along in desired fashion. This is especially helpful for people in sedentary occupations. Try it. Start with the extremities—feet/hands, calves/forearms, thighs/biceps, neck—then move to buttocks, pectorals and abdomen. An occasional stretch is fine while seated or upon rising. Stretch the arms overhead, raise on toes and take a deep breath. (Then shout, laugh, sing, or hum, if possible.) Bend forward with knees straight and stretch out the hamstrings and lower back. (The forward bend with knees clasped is excellent most anytime.) A good yawn or sigh accompanied by a deep breath is also fine most anytime. (Either alone or among understanding friends.) Now and then spend an entire day concentrating on this form of conscious activity. After a whole day it will become quite natural and habitual—and your physical condition will be maintained much better as a result!

General.

A good general rule for anyone to follow is to supplement one's regular exercise routine with "Exercises you aren't built for." Supplementary activities of this kind are best included at some other time of day than during the Daily Dozen, so that more time and concentration can be given to a specific body area, pose or movement. For example, if you desire to work up to a headstand in full lotus position, or do full splits, or work on fairly lengthy yogic breathing techniques, then of course you will need more time than the customary hour it takes to complete the Daily Dozen.

Added to our general rule of practicing "Exercises you aren't built for" are two complementary sub-rules:

(1) The areas of your body that show the most discomfort during exercise are the exact areas that need the most additional work and attention.

(2) The amount of repetitions one repeats an exercise, or whatever type of activity is practiced, will eventually reflect in the size and texture of the muscles and related tissues involved in the activity. For example, you don't see many trapeze artists or long distance runners who look like Sumo wrestlers any more than you would expect Fred Astaire to excel in throwing the hammer or shot-put. Naturally, the individuals who are heavy and slower to begin with, tend to become the weight throwers on the track teams and linemen in football—while the more long and lean types gravitate toward leaping, jumping or running for distances, as in basketball, baseball, track and field events. However, training and practice tend to develop certain physical characteristics.

A case in point would be the muscle types that excel (or are developed) in the course of (or as a result of) types of running events. Sprinters and sprinting require strong bodies that can deliver quick, powerful bursts of speed. The best sprinters will have well developed thighs, buttocks and shoulder muscles. Their endurance is not so much a problem because most sprinter's racing events take less than a minute of concentrated activity. On the other hand a long distance runner is much more in need of stamina and endurance than of power and quickness. He has to carry himself along for miles, so the less bodyweight he carries is all to his advantage. As a result our distance runners tend toward being lean and light and develop further in this direction with lengthy training.

Actually, in later years (if not before) both types would do well to practice the other's specialty part of the time in order to develop an all around body balance. In track and field events the epitome of such body balance is found among decathlon participants, who are required to compete in a varied range of events that are an ultimate test of strength, coordinated jumping and throwing ability, sprinting and distance running—all within a relatively short span of time, which fully tests their stamina and endurance. American decathlon champions such as Bruce Jenner, Bill Toomey, Rafer Johnson, Bob Mathias and Bob Richards exemplify the type of bodies (and men) that result from such a wide range of athletic events and training. Interestingly enough it comes as no great surprise to find that these men, as well as most exceptional athletes, have minds and personalities that compare quite favorably with their physical abilities. But their abilities and accomplishments weren't developed overnight—years of training were involved, usually working hardest at the events they were weakest at in the beginning.

So, if you tend toward being overweight or spreading in some of the usual areas that bulge and broaden as we grow older—or have especially inflexible specific areas—take heart and do more repetitions in the exercises that work upon those particular spots. (Also, walk a lot, "Power Walk," jog/hike, and swim, too, if possible.)

7 Meditation

1. HEAD AND NECK EXERCISES

In addition to their use here as a preparation to meditation, these head and neck exercises were given by Edgar Cayce in numerous instances for people with eye, ear, nose and throat difficulties.

They can be done while sitting straight in a chair with feet flat on the floor, or seated on the ground in "lotus" or "perfect" position (keep hands relaxed, palms upward on the thighs).

Concentrate on keeping the spine straight, the jaw and eyes relaxed, and elongating the neck during the movements. (Eyes may be open or closed as you prefer.)

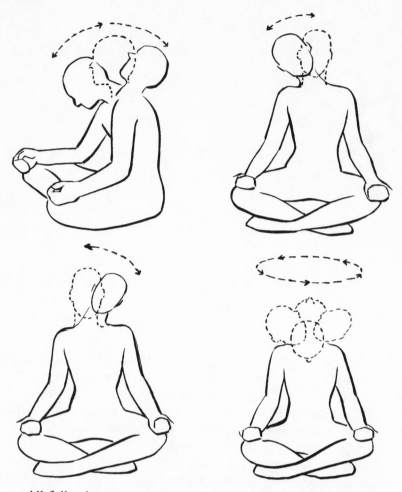

All following movements are repeated three repetitions.

(1) Drop the chin forward (exhaling). Return erect (inhaling).

(2) Raise the chin, head back, elongating the neck and inhaling. Return erect (exhaling).

(3) Drop the right ear to the right, slightly in front of the shoulder. (Do not pivot or twist the neck, but move it as if on a hinge.)

(4) Drop the left ear to the left shoulder (as above).

(5) Drop the chin to the chest (exhaling) then circle to the right a full 360°. Return erect (inhaling).

(6) Reverse the circle movement as above.

    (When done separately it is recommended that these be preceded by a few Egg Rolls and the Cervical Release.)

II. BREATHING

As preparation for meditation
after doing the Head and Neck Exercises

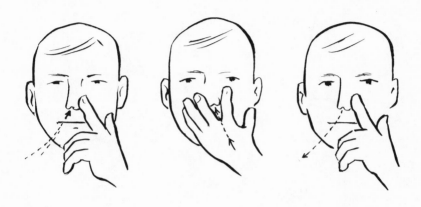

(1) Repeat the affirmation (aloud)—*"Father/Mother God, I will that this activity creates in me a greater channel that Thy will be done."*

(2) Hold the left nostril closed (with left thumb or finger) and breathe in through the right nostril, out of the mouth (three times) affirming:
>   (1) *"In the Name of The Father."*
>   (2) *"In the Name of The Son."*
>   (3) *"In the Name of The Holy Spirit."*

(3) Take three more breaths—in the left nostril and out of the right (holding left forefinger first to right nostril, then left thumb to left nostril) affirming:
>   (1) *"Glory to The Father."*
>   (2) *"Glory to The Son."*
>   (3) *"Glory to The Holy Spirit."*

III. CHANTING
(Three or Seven times)

"Ahhhh—Reeee—Ohmmm" (or any personal chant or mantra one may prefer).

IV. MEDITATION

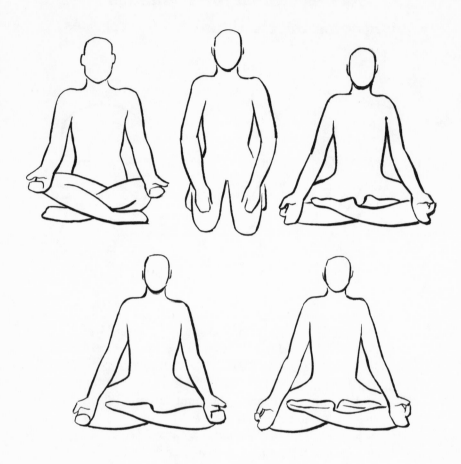

Enter meditation totally relaxed, fixing all thought on "no thought"—or focusing your being on the affirmation, of *"Thy Will Be Done."* If a thought should come, allow it to pass by; don't stay with it. Let it dissolve. Focus the consciousness on the silence of being, the nothingness of thought, on attunement with the universal consciousness. Group meditation may close by joining in the Lord's Prayer as a convening for the group. Individuals may prefer to silently affirm the Lord's Prayer at the beginning or end of meditation. Prayers are, of course, a matter of personal consideration. Meditation will usually last anywhere from five to fifteen minutes, or longer depending on individual preferences. (See: *Journey of Awakening*, by Ram Dass and *Meditation and the Mind of Man*, A.R.E. Press.)

The "Daily Dozen" Extended Routine
(Takes about one hour to complete)

(1) "GOOD MORNING" EXERCISE
(2) JANGLE
(3) SHOULDER SHRUGS
(4) ARM AND LEG CIRCLES
(5) KNEE BENDS ON TOES
(6) "BARNYARD SHUFFLE" LOOSENER
(7) HIP CIRCLES (HULA HOOP)
(8) FORWARD BENDS (KNEES BENT)
(9) EGG ROLL
(10) CERVICAL RELEASE
(11) KNEE AND ELBOW TOUCH
(12) SHOULDER STAND
(13) THE BRIDGE (OR "WHEEL")
(14) THE FISH
(15) LEG RAISES AND SIDE STRETCH
(16) THE CAMEL AND PELVIC STRETCH
(17) SUPINE LAYOUT
(18) THE COBRA
(19) THE LOCUST
(20) THE BOAT
(21) THE BOW

(Break: Having thoroughly arched the spine and exercised the muscle groups involved, we are now ready to move on to some less strenuous loosening activities in a seated position. Now is the time to get up and move around for a minute or two, should you desire to do so.)

(22) YOGA MUDRA (SEATED) AND BELLOWS BREATHING
(23) SHOULDER LOOSENER AND "BALINESE DANCER" MOVEMENT
(24) FACE AND SCALP MASSAGE
(25) ELBOW SQUEEZE
(26) CHEST AND SHOULDER MASSAGE
(27) GROIN AND PELVIC LOOSENING— "STRAIGHT ARROW," BUTTOCKS ROCK, BUTTERFLY, FOOT MASSAGE, GROIN STRETCH MOVEMENTS
(28) JANGLE (PALMS UP)
(29) FLAT-FOOTED SQUATS

(30) KNEE AND GROIN STRENGTHENER
(31) THE CROW
(32) ALTERNATE SIDE BEND AND TOE TOUCH
(33) TIGER STRETCH (WITH VACUUM AND
BUTTOCKS TIGHTENER)

The "Daily Dozen" Short Routine
(Takes about one-half hour to complete)

The short routine is for beginners who are not conditioned physically for the entire routine, or when not enough time is available to complete everything. (The number of repetitions should be determined by the participant according to time and energy available.) Instructions for each exercise follows in Chapter VI.

(1) "GOOD MORNING" EXERCISE
(2) JANGLE
(3) ARM AND LEG CIRCLES
(4) KNEE BENDS (ON TOES)
(5) HULA HOOP
(6) EGG ROLL
(7) CERVICAL RELEASE
(8) KNEE AND ELBOW TOUCH
(9) SHOULDER STAND (OR "THE FISH")
(10) "CAMEL" WITH PELVIC STRETCH (OR
SIDE STRETCH)
(11) REPEAT JANGLE, FLAT FOOTED SQUATS
(12) TIGER STRETCH

The "Daily Dozen": Short Short Routine
(Ten to fifteen minutes to complete)

(1) "GOOD MORNING" EXERCISE
(2) JANGLE
(3) EGG ROLL
(4) CERVICAL RELEASE
(5) TIGER STRETCH

Bibliography And
Recommended References

ANATOMY/PHYSIOLOGY

Gray, Henry (edited by Charles Mayo Gross). *Anatomy of the Human Body*. Philadelphia: Lea & Febiger, 1966. This is the classic medical text, very detailed. Now available in paperback.

Rolf, Ida P., Ph.D. *Rolfing—The Integration of Human Structure*. New York: Harper & Row, 1979. Excellent for its anatomical illustrations and philosophy. A "must" book for all instructors.

The Human Body. New York: Time/Life Books, 1964. A very well presented, easily read and understood explanation of how our bodies are constructed and how they function.

EXERCISE AND YOGA

Cooper, Kenneth H. *Aerobics*. New York: M. Evans, 1968.

Da Liu. *Taoist Health Exercise Book*. New York: Links Books, 1974. Includes Tai Chi Chuan and Reflexology.

Satchidananda, Swami. *Integral Yoga Hatha*. New York: Holt, Rinehart & Winston, 1970. One of the best of all books on hatha yoga.

Stearn, Jess. *Yoga, Youth & Reincarnation*. New York: Bantam Books, 1965. Very good.

Teaching Asanas. Los Altos Hills, California: Ananda Marga Publications, 1973.

Vishnu-devananda, Swami. *The Complete Illustrated Book of Yoga*. New York: Pocket Books, 1972. Also one of the best available on hatha yoga.

MASSAGE AND REFLEXOLOGY

de Langre, Jacques. *The First Book of Do-In*. Hollywood, California: Happiness Press, 1971. The Do-In Book (pronounced "dough-in") owes its allegiance, or rationale, to principles and theories of acupuncture. Excellent diagrams of acupuncture meridians, zone and lymphatic reflex points, along with organic functions and related specific massage. The very best "do-it-yourself" book around. Highly recommended.

Downing, George. *The Massage Book*. New York: Random House, 1972. Probably the best around, includes zone therapy, anatomy charts, massage for lovers, and other valuable information.

MEDITATION

Cayce, Hugh Lynn. *Venture Inward*. New York: Harper & Row, 1964. Excellent.

Dass, Ram. *Journey of Awakening*. New York: Bantam Books, 1978. Put this on your "must read" list. Excellent.

Meditation and the Mind of Man. Virginia Beach: A.R.E. Press, 1975.

Krishna, Gopi. *The Awakening of Kundalini*. New York: E. P. Dutton, 1975.

Naranjo, Claudio and Robert E. Ornstein. *On the Psychology of Meditation*. New York: Viking Press, 1971. This is the best, most scientific treatment of an overview concerning meditation available. Presented by two modern innovative psychologists. Recommended for anyone interested in pursuing the subject.

Search for God, A, Book I. Virginia Beach: A.R.E. Press, 1942. The Edgar Cayce materials add, in a Christianized version of meditation and prayer, most all that Ornstein and Naranjo may have left untouched. Highly recommended for the additional practical information it contains.

Wilhelm, Richard, trans. *The Secret of the Golden Flower*. New York: Harcourt, 1962. Ancient oriental writings on meditation with introductory observations by the eminent psychiatric pioneer, Dr. Carl Jung.

STRESS, PAIN AND SUFFERING

Brown, Barbara B. *Stress and the Art of Biofeedback.* New York: Harper & Row, 1977.

Lamott, Kenneth. *Escape From Stress.* New York: Berkley Windhover, 1975.

Pelletier, Kenneth R., Ph.D. *Mind as Healer/Mind as Slayer: A Holistic Approach to Preventing Stress Disorders.* New York: Delacorte Press, 1977.

Rosa, Karl Robert. *You and AT—Autogenic Training—The Revolutionary Way to Relaxation and Inner Peace.* New York: Saturday Review Press, 1976.

Selye, Hans, M.D. *The Stress of Life.* New York: McGraw Hill, 1976.

Selye, Hans, M.D. *Stress Without Distress.* Philadelphia: Lippincott, 1974.

Shealy, C. Norman, M.D. *Ninety Days to Self Health.* New York: Bantam Books, 1977.

Shealy, C. Norman, M.D. *The Pain Game.* Millbrae, California: Celestial Arts, 1976.

HEALTH AND GENERAL NUTRITION

Adams and Murray. *Body, Mind and the B Vitamins.* New York: Larchmont Books, 1972.

Airola, Paavo O. *Health Secrets From Europe.* New York: Arco Publishing, 1975.

Bolton, Brett. *Edgar Cayce Speaks.* New York: Avon, 1969.

Cott, Allan, M.D., with Jerome Agel and Eugene Boe. *Fasting as a Way of Life.* New York: Bantam Books, 1977.

Fredericks, Carlton. *Psycho-Nutrition.* New York: Grosset & Dunlap, 1976.

Kroeger, Hanna. *Instant Vitamin-Mineral Locator.* Denver: published by author, 1972.

McGarey, William A., M.D. *Edgar Cayce and the Palma Christi.* Virginia Beach: A.R.E. Press, 1967.

Muramoto, Naburo. *Healing Ourselves.* New York: Avon, 1973.

Read, Anne, Carol Ilstrup and Margaret Gammon. *Edgar Cayce on Diet and Health.* New York: Paperback Library, 1969.

Reilly, Harold P. and Ruth Hagy Brod. *The Edgar Cayce Handbook for Health Through Drugless Therapy.* New York: Macmillan, 1975.

Steinhart, Lawrence. *Edgar Cayce Secrets of Beauty Through Health.* New York: Berkley Medallion Books, 1974.

RELATED GENERAL PSYCHOLOGY AND PARAPSYCHOLOGY

Berne, Eric. *Beyond Games and Scripts.* New York: Grove Press, 1976.

Berne, Eric. *Games People Play: The Psychology of Human Relationships.* New York: F. Watts, 1964.

Buscaglia, Leo, Ph.D. *Love.* Thorofare, New Jersey: Charles B. Slack, Inc., 1972.

Dass, Ram, in collaboration with Stephen Levine. *Grist for the Mill.* Santa Cruz, California: Unity Press, 1976. The former Richard Alpert, Ph.D., relates how he went from therapy to therapist, through the psychedelic drug scene and beyond. His search to get it on without drugs. Highly recommended reading.

Dass, Ram. *The Only Dance There Is: Talks Given at the Menninger Foundation, Topeka, Kansas, 1970 and at Spring Grove Hospital, Spring Grove, Maryland, 1972.* Garden City, New York: Anchor Press/Doubleday, 1974.

Dyer, Dr. Wayne W. *Your Erroneous Zones.* New York: Funk & Wagnalls, 1976.

Furst, Jeffrey. *Edgar Cayce's Story of Attitudes and Emotions.* New York: Berkley Books, 1972. This is intended as a workbook for understanding self. Edgar Cayce had a good bit to say on both subjects. We've added some observations from our own experience which we feel tie in well with Cayce's expansive views of human consciousness.

Highest State of Consciousness, The. John White, ed. New York: Doubleday-Anchor, 1972. Editor White has compiled an anthology of highly respected authors and related subjects which dwell upon altered states of consciousness, creativity, psychotherapy, drugs, LSD and mysticism, Transcendental Meditation, meditation and biofeedback, mysticism and schizophrenia, Zen Buddhism, trance and death experiences. The writers span from: D. Ouspensky and the monumental Dr. Richard Maurice Bucke, to modern contributors such as Aldous Huxley, Stanley Krippner, Charles Tart, Richard Wilhelm and Alan Watts. Well worth one's time and consideration.

John, Bubba Free. *The Knee of Listening.* Los Angeles: Dawn Horse Press, 1972.

Keyes, Ken, Jr. *Handbook to Higher Consciousness.* St. Mary, Kentucky: Cornucopia Institute, 1972. Highly worthy of considerable study. Very practical, sound psychological advice, especially for anyone who tends to balk at anything sounding remotely religious, moralistic, preachy or churchish. Excellent thoughts on happiness/unhappiness themes.

Krishna, Gopi. "The True Aim of Yoga," *Psychic Magazine*, Jan./Feb., 1973. Gopi Krishna, an Indian, is founder of The Research Institute for Kundalini. His concise overview of what yoga is and is not, along with observations on meditation, psychic phenomena and the spiritual path, should be required reading for everyone who seriously practices yoga.

Progoff, Ira, Ph.D. *At a Journal Workshop.* New York: Dialogue House Library, 1975.

Steadman, Alice. *Who's the Matter With Me?* Charlotte, North Carolina: CSA Press, 1966.

The Unilaw Library Series

Unilaw Library is a line of inspirational, metaphysical and religious books which demonstrate the basic compatability of classic religious principles with ancient and modern metaphysical cosmology. The line will include fiction, nonfiction, and practical, self-help applications. The purpose of Unilaw Library is to draw from all disciplines which contribute to the evolution of human thought, from the latest scientific discoveries to the re-thinking of old dogmas and attitudes which will lead humanity to the truth about the nature of life and the universe.

If you are interested in other books in the Unilaw series, the following are presently available or coming soon:

Anti-Semitism and Jewish Nationalism
by Jay Pilzer, Ph.D.
A series of essays with introductory passages written by great scholars and philosophers such as Theodor Herzl, Goldwin Smith and H. G. Wells which deal with the emergence of anti-Semitism in pre-World War II Europe, and the consequent development of nationalism leading to the establishment of Israel in 1948. Bibliography.
Softcover $5.95

The Atlanteans—Book I
by David Hyatt
The first in a series of novels in which an American Air Force plane flies through a time-warp and into the city of Poseidia in Atlantis. In this book, the flyers become involved in the struggle between a spiritually-oriented civilization and their materialistic, totalitarian enemy, the sons of Belial.
Softcover $4.95

The Beginning or the End: Where Are We Going?
by The Lusson Twins
Earth changes and lifestyle transitions for the future are presented with guidance for adapting to a new age in this insightful book by remarkable twin psychics. Illustrated.
Hardcover $5.95

Dreams Beyond Dreaming
by Jean Campbell
A fascinating study of dream research, dreaming techniques and the use of dreams to solve problems and help shape one's future.
Hardcover $12.95
Softcover $5.95

Euell Gibbons' Handbook of Edible Wild Plants: A Comprehensive Guide to Identifying and Preparing Edible Wild Plants in the United States and Canada
by Euell Gibbons and Gordon Tucker, Illustrations by Freda Gibbons
A valuable compendium of over 400 edible and palatable plants, over 260 with a drawing for recognizability in the wild. The last book by the internationally known naturalist. Indexed.
Softcover $4.95
Hardcover $9.95

Flee the Wolf! The Story of a Family's Miraculous Journey to Freedom
by Marianne Schmeling

Compelling and autobiographical account of a close-knit family's adaption to life in East Prussia under the Nazi regime, and their flight from the Russians during the closing months of World War II.

Softcover $5.95
Hardcover $9.95

How To Live Creatively
by Dorothy Evelyn Stanley, Ph.D.

A series of lectures on the way thinking creates real events. Attitudes and emotions, how to deal with grief, the secret of staying young, and other subjects.

Softcover $4.95

Life Signs: An Astrological Casebook
by Mary Jones and Dan Fry

An astrologer for over 25 years, Fry demonstrates, using meticulously documented histories of real people and real events, that through scientific mathematical computation of the position of the planets, trends and influences upon people's lives can be accurately determined and interpreted. Illustrated with charts.

Softcover $4.95

The Mark Twain Proposition
by Gina Cerminara

First novel by the author of the best-selling *Many Mansions* takes a witty, humorous, and highly intelligent look at race prejudice in America. In its second printing.

Softcover $4.95

New Life Cookbook: Based on the Health and Nutritional Philosophy of the Edgar Cayce Readings
by Marceline A. Newton, Introduction by Hugh Lynn Cayce

Over 400 recipes developed from Cayce's dietary recommendations present a simplified, practical approach to high-fiber, naturally delicious meals. In its third printing. Indexed.

Softcover $4.95

The Over-29 Health Book: A Unique Approach to Exercise and Well-Being Based Upon the Philosophical Concepts in Yoga and the Edgar Cayce Readings
by Jeffrey Furst, Introduction by C. Norman Shealy, M.D.

The only exercise book dealing with the lymphatic system, attacking the basic cause of illness through the use of exercise (the "Daily Dozen") to facilitate the removal of toxic wastes from the body and to supply the cells and tissues with the nutrients and oxygen they need. Illustrated and bibliography.

Softcover $5.95

The Parable: A Story of Jesus, Son of Joseph
by Cleta Flynn

A narrative re-creation, derived from a variety of sources, of Yeshua ben

Josephus (Jesus son of Joseph) in his thirteenth year, presenting him as what he himself claimed to be: a prophet, a spokesman for Yahweh, God, to his people, Israel.

Softcover $4.95
Hardcover $7.95

The Renderings of Stefanos: Book I—Science and Technology
by Stefan Grunwald, Ph.D.

First of a series of books channeled through a university professor in a trance state. This book concerns a psychoanalysis of humanity vis-a-vis the development and use of science and technology, and the manner in which it has led to a scientifically-inspired rape of the earth's resources. Includes detailed question and answer sessions posed by scientists and an introduction covering the fascinating story of how a man totally ignorant and skeptical of psychic phenomena became an altered-consciousness psychic.

Softcover $4.95

Starborn: A Mystical Tale
by John Nelson

Humorous metaphysical novel about a baby mistakenly born with his cosmic memory intact, and a misguided child psychologist who attempts to recruit him for her crusade to train psychic children to take over the world and make it safe for humanity.

Softcover $4.95

The Vedanta of Pure Non-Dualism
Translated by I. C. Sharma, Ph.D.

The first translation of the great religious thinker, Sri Vallabhacharya, a contemporary of Martin Luther, and founder of a Hindu movement with over a hundred million followers and a 500-year history.

Softcover $4.95
Hardcover $9.95

Very Practical Meditation
by Serene West

The first practical guide to using meditation for specific end results, such as overcoming fear, boredom, anxiety, etc., along with instructions to learn effective meditation.

Softcover $4.95

To order, enclose check or money order, payable to Donning Publishers, for price of books, plus $.75 shipping for one book, $.25 for each additional book. Virginia residents add 4% sales tax.

To order, enclose check or money order, payable to Donning Publishers, for price of books, plus $.75 shipping for one book, $.25 for each additional book. Virginia residents add 4% sales tax.

Send to: The Donning Company/Publishers
5659 Virginia Beach Blvd.
Norfolk, VA 23502